Cholesterol Lowering
A practical guide to therapy

Edited by

Jonathan Abrams MD
Professor of Medicine, Division of Cardiology
University of New Mexico Health Service Center,
Albuquerque, New Mexico

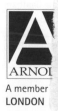

ARNOL

A member
LONDON

First published in Great Britain in 2003 by
Arnold, a member of the Hodder Headline Group,
338 Euston Road, London NW1 3BH

http://www.arnoldpublishers.com

Distributed in the United States of America by
Oxford University Press Inc.,
198 Madison Avenue, New York, NY10016
Oxford is a registered trademark of Oxford University Press

Whilst the advice and information in this book are believed to be true and
accurate at the date of going to press, neither the authors nor the publisher
can accept any legal responsibility or liability for any errors or omissions
that may be made. In particular (but without limiting the generality of the
preceding disclaimer) every effort has been made to check drug dosages;
however, it is still possible that errors have been missed. Furthermore,
dosage schedules are constantly being revised and new side-effects
recognized. For these reasons the reader is strongly urged to consult the
drug companies' printed instructions before administering any of the drugs
recommended in this book.

British Library Cataloguing in Publication Data
A catalogue record for this book is available from the British Library

Library of Congress Cataloging-in-Publication Data
A catalog record for this book is available from the Library of Congress

ISBN 0 340 76132 6

1 2 3 4 5 6 7 8 9 10

Commissioning Editor: Joanna Koster
Development Editor: Sarah Burrows
Project Editor: Wendy Rooke
Production Controller: Deborah Smith
Cover Design: Lee-May Lim

Typeset in 10 on 12 pt Minion by Phoenix Photosetting, Chatham, Kent
Printed and bound in Malta

What do you think about this book? Or any other Arnold title?
Please send your comments to feedback.arnold@hodder.co.uk

Contents

Contributors

Jonthan Abrams, MD
Division of Cardiology, University of New Mexico Health Service Center, Albuquerque, NM, USA

Bradford C Berk, MD
Chief, Cardiology Division, University of Rochester Medical Center, Rochester, NY, USA

Jerome D Cohen, MD
Division of Cardiology, St. Louis University Health Sciences Center, St Louis, MO, USA

Donald B Hunninghake
Director, Heart Disease Prevention Clinic, University of Minnesota Medical School, Minneapolis, Minnesota, USA

Michael D Klein, MD
Cardiology Department, Boston Medical Center, Boston, MA, USA

Robert H Knopp, MD
Director, Northwest Lipid Research Clinic, and Professor of Medicine, University of Washington School of Medicine, Seattle, Washington, USA

Judith R McNamara
Lipid Research Laboratory, Lipid and Heart Disease Prevention Program; and
Division of Endocrinology, Metabolism, Diabetes & Molecular Medicine, New England Medical Center, Tufts University School of Medicine, Boston MA, USA

Merle Myerson, MD, EdD
Division of Cardiology, College of Physicians and Surgeons, Columbia University, New York, NY, USA

Richard C Pasternak, MD, FACC
Cardiology Division, Massachusetts General Hospital, Boston, MA, USA

Sanjeev Puri, MD
Division of Cardiology, University of Arkansas Medical Center, Little Rock, AK, USA

Ernst J Schaefer, MD
Lipid Research Laboratory, Lipid and Heart Disease Prevention Program; and
Division of Endocrinology, Metabolism, Diabetes & Molecular Medicine, New England Medical Center, Tufts University School of Medicine, Boston MA, USA

Leo J Seman
Lipid Research Laboratory, Lipid and Heart Disease Prevention Program; and

Division of Endocrinology, Metabolism, Diabetes & Molecular Medicine, New England Medical Center, Tufts University School of Medicine, Boston MA, USA. Current address: Bayer Corp., West Haven, CT, USA

Neil J Stone, MD
Professor of Clinical Medicine (Cardiology), Northwestern University School of Medicine, Chicago, IL, USA

Sylvia Vela, MD
Division of Endocrinology, Carl T. Hayden VA Medical Center, Phoenix, AZ, USA

Daniel A Wuthrich, MD
Department of Medicine, Division of Cardiology, University of Washington, Seattle, WA, USA

Foreword

Cholesterol Lowering is a comprehensive and valuable description of the advance made during the past decade in the diagnosis and management of hypercholesterolemia. The book is well researched, is authored by authoritative scholars and opinion leaders, and deals with the most significant issues of clinical and scientific interest concerning cholesterol metabolism and its relationship to coronary heart disease. The book goes from the basic to the bedside. It describes the carriers of cholesterol, the lipoproteins, their relationship to atherosclerosis, and their role in regulating lipid metabolism. It discusses the causes of hypercholesterolemia translated into hyperlipoproteinemia, both primary and secondary. It discusses issues of diagnosis, of what to measure, of whom to treat, and how to treat with therapeutic lifestyle intervention and drugs. A great deal of emphasis is placed on events of the past decade, which include six epic trials with statins that show a remarkable degree of consistency. Relative risk reduction varied from 24 to 37 percent for major cardiovascular events, despite the fact that the studies were carried out with three different statins and in six different populations in different parts of the world, both in primary and secondary prevention. This is a remarkable degree of consistency which provides support for a class effect of statins in reducing the burden of coronary heart disease. *Cholesterol Lowering* also emphasizes the guidelines for the management of cholesterol, the most recent version of which – NCEP-ATPIII – were published in 2001. Despite the enormous amount of information showing the benefit of lifestyle management and of statin therapy in the treatment and prevention of coronary heart disease, all currently available evidence points to a vast under-diagnosis and under-treatment. With the current guidelines, at least 36 million Americans could benefit by therapy, yet only about one-third of this number are treated. Of those patients who begin treatment, the number who persist is disappointingly small. One lesson that we learned from the AFCAPS/TexCAPS study is that one of the strongest inducers of taking a statin is actually to have an event – but this is a hard way to get a message across. One-and-a-half to two years after AFCAPS/TexCAPS was completed, approximately 85 percent of the participants who had experienced a primary coronary event during the course of the study were taking a statin – a remarkable finding. If we could find some way to impart the message to the at-risk population to influence this degree of behavior change and its persistence over a two-year period, this indeed would be a remarkable achievement. This book presents an important addition to armamentarium of the clinician, scholar, investigator and student of lipid disorders, cholesterol metabolism and coronary disease.

Antonio M. Gotto, Jr, MD, DPhil
The Stephen and Suzanne Weiss Dean
Joan and Sanford I. Weill Medical College of Cornell University
New York, NY, USA

Preface

This monograph has a modest goal: to outline and interpret the basic facts about lipid disorders and their treatment. The results of a large number of important randomized clinical trials have been published over the past decade that unequivocally confirm the 'cholesterol hypothesis' – that is, that an abnormal lipid profile or dyslipidemia imparts an increased risk for the development of cardiovascular disease. Furthermore, effective drug therapy for lipid disorders has been repeatedly demonstrated to lower cardiovascular risk, with reductions in both coronary artery disease and stroke.

Cholesterol Lowering deals with lipid physiology; how to assay lipid components; and the relationship of dyslipidemia to other medical disorders (secondary dyslipidemia). The basic science underpinning the cholesterol hypothesis is provided in a clear manner. Dietary measures and pharmacological approaches are presented in detail. Finally, a 'for whom' and 'how to' approach should allay the uncertainties of clinicians and provide a clear road map to diagnosis and therapy.

Jonathan Abrams
2003

1

Current rationale for lipid lowering

JONATHAN ABRAMS

Over the past decade there has been a veritable revolution in our understanding of hypercholesterolemia and its effect on clinical coronary artery disease (CAD). Although a large amount of information has been available for years regarding the adverse consequences of abnormal lipid levels in animals and humans, along with considerable epidemiological evidence that has underscored the health hazards of hyperlipidemia, the cholesterol controversy has long remained a subject of discord, disagreement, and denial for many. While a number of controversies and unresolved issues remain (see Box 1.1), it now is incontrovertible that for individuals with established CAD, or high-risk 'primary prevention' subjects, lowering of total elevated and particularly low-density lipoprotein (LDL) or LDL cholesterol (LDL-C) prolongs survival and decreases cardiovascular morbidity.[1-5] Furthermore, favorable changes in high-density lipoprotein (HDL) cholesterol (HDL-C) and triglyceride also decrease CAD[6-7] events. This discussion will summarize recent clinical data that provide the basis for our current view that aggressive lipid lowering in selective individuals is imperative, and no longer just one of several treatment options for the patient with CAD.

THE OLD DATA

Many clinical trials, guidelines and expert panel recommendations over the past decade have suggested that lipid lowering provides a survival advantage for individuals with high baseline total and LDL-C. It is also clear that low levels of HDL

Box 1.1 *Cholesterol: some remaining controversies*

- Is LDL-cholesterol the best target versus non-HDL-cholesterol?
- Should LDL particle size (pattern A versus B) make a difference in drug selection?
- Is hypertriglyceridemia an independent risk factor deserving treatment?
- How low should LDL be reduced? Should there be different target goals for subjects at differing risk?
- Is there a cut-off point below which LDL therapy is unnecessary?
- Should post-prandial lipid levels be used as a guide to selection of therapy?
- Is a low HDL a legitimate independent target for drug therapy?
- Are there long-term adverse health consequences with statin use?
- How important are the non-lipid or pleotropic actions of the statins?

or HDL-C impact independent risk for CAD, although there are as yet no clinical trial data available to confirm a benefit solely from raising HDL-C; nor are agents yet available that target HDL without affecting triglyceride levels. Hypertriglyceridemia, which remains the subject of some controversy, is a contributory adverse factor, especially in the presence of an elevated LDL-C, and perhaps as the sole lipid abnormality in some patients.[8-10] Furthermore, low HDL-C by itself contributes to increased morbidity and mortality.[6,7,11,12]

In spite of the large amount of older observational data relating to the benefits of achieving low total and LDL-C levels, until relatively recently many experts and physicians remained unimpressed by the cholesterol hypothesis. In retrospect, a major problem with past studies was the relative inefficiency of the older cholesterol-lowering modalities (e.g. diet, fibrates, and resins). Most older intervention trials provided a reduction of no more than 10–15 percent in total and LDL-C. In the landmark 7-year LRC CCPT (Lipid Research Clinics Coronary Primary Prevention Trial) using a bile acid or resin agent, LDL was lowered by 12.6 percent, although in individuals who were compliant with cholestyramine, reduction in LDL was often much more impressive.[13] Meta-analyses have indicated that the benefits of lipid lowering are in direct proportion to the degree of decrease in total and cholesterol and LDL.[14-16] Most earlier interventions, of modest hypolipidemic effectiveness, have been only suggestively positive or inconclusive. Another factor impeding acceptance of the cholesterol hypothesis was the failure to demonstrate a reduction in total or all-cause mortality in early published trials. Finally, the possible risks of lowering cholesterol as well as concerns about serious adverse consequences of pharmacological intervention, slowed acceptance of a vigorous cholesterol-lowering policy.

The pre-statin era trials that have been considered as positive evidence for lipid-lowering efficacy were carried out during the 1980s. The results, while supportive of cholesterol lowering, were not dramatic; furthermore, most of the available therapies were not easy for patients to utilize. This is obviously true for the POSCH (Ileal Bypass Trial), which in reality provided powerful evidence in support of the cholesterol hypothesis.[17] Through a series of reports, all of which confirmed an increasing benefit from reductions in cholesterol over many years, the POSCH trial[17,18] in effect predicted the positive results of the statin era randomized clinical trials.[1–5,14–16]

In conclusion, the older clinical trial data, while generally concordant with epidemiological studies and considerable basic science and animal research,[19] did not convince most clinicians in the United States and elsewhere that cholesterol lowering is valuable. The chorus of naysaying and controversy, coupled with questionable validity of available data, promoted a considerable degree of uncertainty among the lay public as well as the medical profession. All of this rapidly changed after November, 1994, when the results of the landmark Scandinavian Simvastatin Survival Study (4S) were reported (see Appendix),[1] followed by Western Scotland in 1995,[4] CARE in 1996,[2] AFCAPS,[5] and LIPID,[3] in 1998.

THE NEW VASCULAR BIOLOGY

An important component of our current understanding of the adverse impact of hyperlipidemia has come from a large body of evidence relating to the biology and pathophysiology of the vascular wall and the impact of elevated LDL-C on the function and patho-anatomy of the coronary arteries (see Chapter 2). A variety of arterial wall phenomena that adversely affect coronary artery function and physiology, and are directly related to elevated LDL-C, oxidized LDL, or other dyslipidemias, are under intense investigation. Thus, a robust body of research over the past decade extends our knowledge and understanding of the consequences of hyperlipidemia on the vessel wall.[20] While new therapies will ultimately become available that will favorably affect atherosclerosis, at the present time LDL-C lowering is the most effective way to improve coronary vascular function and the propensity for atherogenesis, smooth muscle proliferation, and the inflammatory responses now recognized to be a part of the atherosclerotic process.[20–23] Although the anti-oxidant hypothesis is scientifically attractive, currently available clinical trial data do not support the view that administration of exogenous anti-oxidants will provide additional benefits over and above effective lipid lowering.[24–26]

Endothelial dysfunction

Perturbations of endothelial function involve a variety of phenomena that adversely affect the vessel wall, and ultimately lead to atherogenesis and cellular proliferation. The most carefully studied endothelial abnormality of the vasculature is that of vasomotor function. Animal studies and a variety of human investigations have now shown conclusively that dyslipidemia – and particularly elevated LDL-C – is associated with disordered arterial vasodilator responses to a variety of stimuli.[27–34] Thus, coronary atherosclerosis that is mild to severe, or even hypercholesterolemia in the absence of angiographic evidence of coronary plaque, are associated with impaired vasodilator responses in the coronary and systemic circulations, consonant with endothelial vasomotor dysfunction of large and small arteries. The classic experimental approach in such investigations is to infuse acetylcholine (ACh) into a coronary artery and then assess the vasodilator/vasoconstrictor responses of the vessel. Normally, ACh stimulates a receptor that triggers guanylate cyclase activation induced by formation and release of nitric oxide (NO) within the endothelial cell, resulting in smooth muscle vasorelaxation. In healthy vessels, ACh and other endothelial-dependent stimuli (e.g. exercise, shear stress) induce vasodilation. However, in the presence of endothelial dysfunction, often related to the reduced availability of NO, arterial vasodilator responses may be blunted, and even constrictor in nature (Figure 1.1). In essence, a physiological or exogenous stimulus that normally evokes arterial dilatation may induce a decreased degree of dilatation or even overt vasoconstriction.[27-34]

In the presence of endothelial function, coronary vessels are more likely to constrict at focal sites of impaired NO availability. Furthermore, such vessels may not be able to enlarge to a normal degree in response to vasodilator stimuli, such as exercise. Coronary flow reserve may be impaired, indicating that the coronary resistance vessels also demonstrate disordered vasodilator activity.[30] These abnormalities may have relevance to the precipitation of ischemic episodes, both painful (angina) and silent.

The multiple mechanisms whereby hypercholesterolemia affects the endothelium are being actively investigated (see Chapter 2). One common hypothesis relates to increased oxygen free radical production in endothelial and vascular smooth muscle cells. NO is degraded more rapidly and completely in the presence of this oxidant stress. Oxidation of LDL-C (LDL-OX) is related to this process.[20-23] In the setting of elevated LDL or LDL-OX, endothelial function in angiographically normal coronary arteries, as well as atherosclerotic vessels, is abnormal (see Figure 1.1)[27-30]; there is a greater propensity for vasoconstriction or impaired vasodilatation to stimuli that normally induce dilation of the arteries (e.g. exercise, mental stress, cold pressor testing).

The good news is the now well-documented observation that reduction in LDL-C may restore or improve the baseline endothelial dysfunction demonstrable in hypercholesterolemia or in diseased coronary arteries, resulting in enhanced dilator responses and less vasoconstriction (Figure 1.1). This improvement has been demonstrated in large epicardial coronary conduit vessels, typically involved in the atherosclerotic process,[28-34] as well as the coronary microcirculation. The latter are coronary arterioles or smaller vessels which modulate coronary blood flow, and are in part responsible for the impaired coronary reserve common to individuals with typical CAD.[30] One study suggested that LDL-C may have to be significantly elevated for starting therapy in order to improve coronary vasomotor responses.[28] Limited data indicate that ambulatory myocardial ischemia may be reduced in patients with CAD who are hyperlipidemic following treatment with potent LDL-C-lowering drugs; that is, the statins.[35,36] It is thus reasonable to recommend that such agents should be part of the routine medical therapy of dyslipidemic patients with proven CAD and angina or those who have had a prior myocardial infarction. The existing clinical trial database supports such a recommendation (see below, Appendix). In the large randomized clinical trials (RCT), rates of angina pectoris have been substantially reduced,[1,26] and in all, the need for coronary revascularization was decreased.[1-5,26] These data strongly support favorable effects on the decreased coronary circulation. Furthermore, the Heart Protection Study (HPS) suggests that baseline LDL-C need not be elevated to achieve benefit in subjects at increased

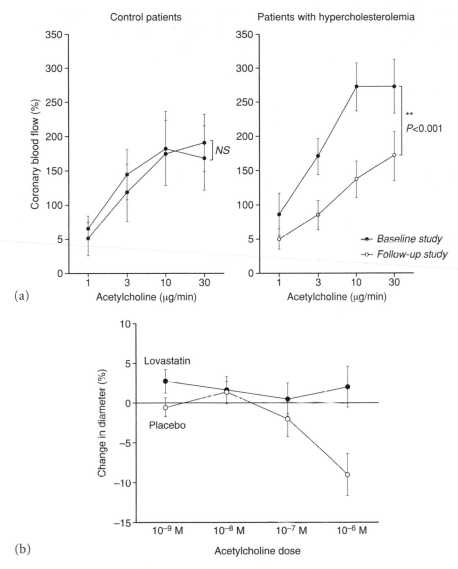

Figure 1.1 *(a) Coronary blood flow responses to acetylcholine (ACh) in resistance vessels of the coronary circulation. Left: responses of patients with coronary atherosclerosis and normal cholesterol before and after pravastatin therapy for 6 months; no improvement was seen. Right: comparable coronary artery disease (CAD) subjects but with hypercholesterolemia demonstrate a robust response to prevastatin, with markedly enhanced coronary blood flow responses to ACh. In this study, enhanced vasodilation of the epicardial coronary vessels was also demonstrated in the hypercholesterolemic group following 6 months of pravastatin treatment (data not shown). Reproduced from Reference 30. (b) Data representing ACh responses in hypercholesterolemic subjects with CAD before and after 6 months of lovastatin therapy, or placebo. The upper curve indicates improved vasodilator capacity to ACh after 6 months of cholesterol lowering with lovastatin. The baseline data are not presented, but the two groups of patients had comparable degrees of vasoconstriction to ACh before the treatment periods. Reproduced from Reference 31.*

vascular risk, even those without overt coronary or cerebrovascular disease.[26] Thus, in several thousand diabetics free of clinical vascular events, there was a robust risk reduction that was equivalent to all cohorts in the study.

Atherogenesis

In Chapter 2, Drs Wuthrich and Berk review the basic mechanisms by which atherosclerosis is initiated and progresses. Monocytes and activated lymphocytes are part of the process; it is now recognized that atherogenesis is in part an inflammatory condition.[37-39] Adhesion molecule expression is facilitated by elevated LDL-C. Infiltration of the intima by LDL particles – particularly modified or oxidized LDL – is part of the atherosclerotic process. Significant reductions in LDL and oxidized LDL-C result in a less 'activated' vessel wall with a decreased propensity for inflammation and atherosclerosis.

Biology of the atherosclerotic plaque

A major advance in our understanding of CAD over the past decade has been the recognition that atherosclerotic plaques or lesions demonstrate a wide variability in their composition: susceptibility to injury, ulceration, or fissuring; degree of fibrosis and calcification; and propensity to initiate 'plaque events' that may result in intramural, mural, or obstructive thrombotic phenomena. A large body of previous and current research is devoted to plaque biology and characteristics, including those phenomena that may predispose to plaque rupture, fissuring, or erosion. Some of the factors that are associated with an increased propensity of plaques to ulcerate or rupture are listed in Box 1.2.

Many of these characteristics may be favorably modified by lipid lowering, particularly decreases in LDL and oxidized LDL. Thus, *vulnerable* or *unstable* atherosclerotic plaque may be converted to *protected* or *stable* plaque. Lesions that are less prone to injury, ulceration or fissuring are clearly 'safer' and result in fewer clinical and sub-clinical atherosclerotic events. Cholesterol esters in the necrotic core of the plaque are decreased by lowering of LDL. Plaque stabilization helps explain the remarkable benefits of the lipid lowering that has been well documented in recent clinical trials in CAD patients using the HMG-CoA reductase inhibitors.[1-3,26,40-42]

Box 1.2 *Some important characteristics of vulnerable plaque*

- Thin fibrous cap
- Lipid–rich plaque (often with necrotic core)
- Marked inflammatory process, usually maximal at shoulder of plaque
- Expression of matrix metalloproteinases
- Poor smooth muscle content within plaque
- Adventitial inflammatory cell activation

THE REMARKABLE SUCCESS STORY OF LIPID LOWERING

Although the epidemiological and clinical trial data of the past 20–30 years convinced many that the 'Cholesterol Hypothesis' is valid, firm evidence that aggressive efforts to decrease total and LDL-C has been late in coming. Controversy has swirled around this issue, with confusion and uncertainty coloring the view of many. As mentioned, several factors have contributed to this state of affairs:

1. The potency of traditional lipid-lowering interventions – diet, resins, fibrates – is modest and often disappointing.
2. Total or all-cause mortality was not lowered in the early trials, although CAD events and mortality were often favorably affected in the intervention group.
3. The suggestion of possible harm related to cholesterol lowering was quite influential, with some suggesting that subjects randomized to active lipid drug therapy may have an increase in cancer, suicide, or violent death.

In addition to the robust contribution of vascular biology (see Chapter 2) to the emerging story favoring lipid lowering, two major lines of evidence have demonstrated convincingly that lowering total and LDL-C in high-risk individuals with and without vascular disease substantially decreases CAD morbidity and mortality: (1) the aggregate experience from a variety of coronary and carotid artery regression trials[18,43–48]; and (2) the dramatic decreases in major coronary events in the six large lipid-lowering trials reported since 1994 (Figure 1.2; see Appendix).[1–6,26] These studies, which deal with primary and secondary prevention populations, have consistently produced striking and consistent benefits, including a decrease in total or all-cause mortality in some trials.[1,3,4,26] The relative risk reductions for various clinical events achieved in the first five major randomized statin clinical trials (RCT) are indicated in Figure 1.2. The magnitude of reduction of baseline total and LDL-C in these studies is significantly greater than that achieved in any prior lipid intervention trials; the marked reduction in LDL is the key to the remarkable RCT results that have accumulated since 1994. Lowering triglyceride levels and raising HDL-C are likely to contribute to the beneficial outcomes.[6,7]

Advent of the HMG CoA reductase inhibitors or statins

The pharmacology of these potent drugs is discussed by Dr Hunninghake in Chapter 8. In brief, these agents interfere with cholesterol synthesis in hepatic cells, and induce up-regulation of LDL-receptors on the cell surface. It is now accepted that the statin drugs have important non-lipid actions (pleiotropic effects) in addition to lowering of total and LDL-C.[49–51] These agents also decrease triglycerides and modestly increase HDL-C; nevertheless, it is assumed that the dramatic reduction in LDL-C produced by the statins is primarily responsible for the robust success of the regression studies and cardiovascular event trials employing a statin. The ability to lower total cholesterol reliably by 20–30 percent, and LDL-C by 25–40 percent, has provided physicians with a remarkably potent tool to favorably affect the natural history of atherosclerosis. Furthermore, modest increases in HDL-C more than likely contribute to the clinical benefits of the statins. Many believe that the total

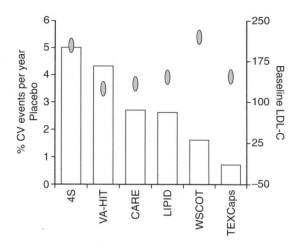

Figure 1.2 *Cardiovascular (CV) death and non-fatal myocardial infarction in major lipid randomized controlled trials (RCT).*

cholesterol to HDL-C ratio (TC/HDL) is the most useful predictor of cardiac events; the HMG-CoA reductase inhibitors favorably affect both the numerator and the denominator of this ratio.

Consistent reductions in non-fatal myocardial infarction, unstable angina, cardiovascular death, revascularization rates, and stroke have been the most noteworthy findings of these reports.[1–5,26] In the aggregate, the regression trial experience predicted and has amplified the series of large RCTs of lipid lowering with the HMG-CoA reductase inhibitors (see Appendix; Figure 1.2).[18,26,43–48] The findings of two recent trials, AVERT[40] and MIRACL,[41] as well those of a Swedish[52] and a German[42] report, suggest benefits of aggressive lipid lowering to reductions in non-fatal events in patients with stable and unstable angina as well as acute myocardial infarction. Other data are supportive for the initiation of statin therapy early in acute coronary syndromes.[53] Observational analysis suggests that patients on a statin at the time of percutaneous intervention (PCI) have an improved survival at 30 days and 6 months after PCI, compared to subjects who were not receiving statins at the time of the PCI. Finally, VA-HIT, employing the fibric acid agent gemfibrozil to raise HDL-C and lower triglycerides, demonstrated a substantial clinical event benefit in older males with CAD, normal LDL-C, and low HDL-C.[7]

Thus, current appreciation of the value of lipid lowering is derived primarily from the remarkable series of large statin trials, all of which demonstrated concordant clinical benefits beginning within 2–3 years of initiation of therapy (Figure 1.3; see Appendix). Following 4S (1994),[1] which enrolled the highest risk patients of all the studies, two more secondary prevention trials, CARE (1996)[2] and LIPID (1998),[3] were reported that enlarged the database and broadened the indications for statin therapy in a variety of patient cohorts with CAD. All three studies demonstrated robust and concordant decreases in cardiovascular morbidity and mortality. In

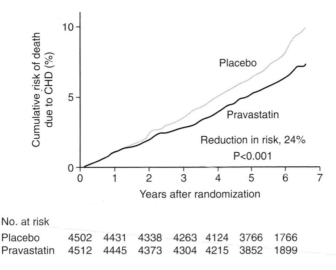

Figure 1.3 *Event curves for pravastatin and placebo in the CARE trial, a post-infarction lipid lowering study. Note that the curves do not begin to separate for 1–2 years; virtually all of the major statin trials have shown the same phenomenon, with late protection against vascular events in stable patients. The protection from statins may indeed occur earlier in acute coronary syndrome subjects. From reference 2; see also appendix.*

addition, the small but positive Post-CABG Trial was reported in 1997.[47] Western Scotland[4] and TEXCaps-AFCaps[5] demonstrated similar benefits in high- and low-risk healthy populations with dyslipidemia (primary prevention), respectively. More recently, the results of the huge Heart Protection Study (HPS) were reported.[26] HPS is by far the largest lipid-lowering trial to date, and the objective was to enroll high-risk individuals for major vascular events, most – but not all – of whom at entry had established vascular disease. An additional objective was to determine whether simvastatin and/or an antioxidant vitamin 'cocktail' would reduce cardiovascular risk, irrespective of baseline lipid values (see also Appendix). A total of 21 536 subjects was enrolled, including large numbers of elderly (aged 65–80 years) men and women. A relative risk reduction of 24 percent was seen for virtually all subjects of individuals at high risk. Diabetics without overt vascular disease also benefited, as did those with baseline LDL-C levels under 100 mg/dL. The antioxidant vitamin mixture had a neutral effect on all endpoints.

Thus, over 55 000 subjects have been randomized to placebo or statin (simvastatin, lovastatin, pravastatin) in the six major RCTs.[1–5,26] The degree of LDL and total cholesterol reduction has been comparable in each study, and even greater in the two small high-dose atorvastatin studies (AVERT, MIRACL).[40,41] While the study population baseline cardiovascular risk is quite different among the various trials, the clinical event benefits are comparable and remarkably consistent (see Figure 1.2 and Appendix). The Appendix contains condensed summaries of the six large statin RCTs, as well as details of AVERT, MIRACL, HATS, and VA-HIT; HATS is a small regression study employing niacin in combination with simvastatin.[54]

CONCLUSIONS

While the baseline cardiovascular risk in the large statin RCT ranges from very high (4S) to very low (TEXCaps), the degree of risk reduction in clinical endpoints is remarkably similar among the studies (Figure 1.2; Appendix). The mean age, sex ratio, and percentage of diabetics in the trials vary considerably among the different trials; nevertheless, the concordance of all important endpoint reductions in diabetics, women, and older subjects, indicates a broad-based benefit for most patients with dyslipidemia. The VA-HIT study confirms an important benefit with gemfibrozil in males with CAD, low HDL, normal LDL, and high triglycerides.[7] AVERT,[41] MIRACL[42] and HATS each provide additional support for importance of aggressive therapy of dyslipidemia in CAD subjects. HPS potentially broadens the population for statin treatment to much lower risk subjects than previously reported.[26]

Finally, the debate as to whether aggressive treatment of high cholesterol or dyslipidemia decreases morbidity and mortality is no longer relevant. Robust reductions in CAD mortality, non-fatal infarction, stroke, and need for revascularization have been repeatedly documented in the statin trials as well as the VA-HIT study.[1–5,7,26] **The cholesterol hypothesis has been proven**; now, the medical community must strive to make statins, niacin – as well as the fibrates – available to all appropriate subjects. The Heart Protection Study suggests that a statin may be beneficial in patients at high risk who have normal or low baseline LDL levels.[26]

REFERENCES

1. Scandinavian Simvastatin Survival Study Group. Randomized trial of cholesterol lowering in 4444 patients with coronary heart disease: The Scandinavian Simvastatin Survival Study (4S). *Lancet* 1994; **344**: 1383–9.
2. Sacks FM, Pfeffer MA, Moye LA, *et al.* The effect of pravastatin on coronary events after myocardial infarction in patients with average cholesterol levels. *N Engl J Med* 1996; **335**: 1001–9.
3. The Long-Term Intervention with Pravastatin in Ischemic Heart Disease (LIPID) Study Group. Prevention of cardiovascular events and death with pravastatin in patients with coronary heart disease and a broad range of initial cholesterol levels. *N Engl J Med* 1998; **339**: 1349–57.
4. Shepard J, Cobbe SM, Ford I, *et al.* Prevention of coronary heart disease with pravastatin in men with hypercholesterolemia. *N Engl J Med* 1995; **333**: 1301–7.
5. Downs JR, Clearfield M, Wiess S, *et al.* Primary prevention of acute coronary events with lovastatin in men and women with average cholesterol levels: results of AFCAPS/TEXCaps. *JAMA* 1998; **279**: 1615–22.
6. Frick MH, Elo O, Haapa K, *et al.* Helsinki Heart Study: primary prevention trial with gemfibrozil in middle-aged men with dyslipidemia. *N Engl J Med* 1987; **317**: 1237–45.
7. Rubins HB, Robins SJ, Iwane MK, *et al.* Gemfibrozil for the secondary prevention of coronary heart disease in men with low levels of high-density lipoprotein cholesterol. *N Engl J Med* 1999; **341**: 410–18.

8. Austin MA. Plasma triglycerides and coronary heart disease. *Arterioscler Thromb* 1991; **11**: 2–14.

9. Ginsberg HN. Is hypertriglyceridemia a risk factor for atherosclerotic disease? A simple question with a complicated answer. *Ann Intern Med* 1997; **126**: 912–14.

10. Austin MA, Hokansen JE, Edwards KL. Hyperlipidemia as a cardiovascular risk factor. *Am J Cardiol* 1998; **81**: 7B–12B.

11. Gordon DJ, Probstfield JL, Garrison RJ, *et al*. High-density lipoprotein cholesterol and cardiovascular disease: four prospective American Studies. *Circulation* 1989; **79**: 8–15.

12. Von Eckardstein A, Assmann G. Prevention of coronary heart disease by raising high-density lipoprotein cholesterol. *Curr Opin Lipidol* 2000; **11**: 627–37.

13. Lipid Research Clinics Program. The Lipid Research Clinics Coronary Primary Prevention Trial results. 1. Reduction in incidence of coronary heart disease. *JAMA* 1984; **251**: 351–64; Part II: pp. 365–74.

14. Ross SD, Allen IE, Connelly JE, *et al*. Clinical outcomes in statin treatment trials – A meta-analysis. *Arch Intern Med* 1999; **159**: 1793–802.

15. LaRosa JC, He J, Vupputuri S. Effect of statins on risk of coronary disease: a meta-analysis of randomized controlled trials. *JAMA* 1999; **282**: 2340–6.

16. Auer J, Berent R, Eber B. Lessons learned from statin trials. *Clin Cardiol* 2001; **24**: 277–80.

17. Buchwald H, Varco RL, Matts JP, *et al*. Effect of partial ileal bypass surgery on mortality and morbidity from coronary heart disease in patients with hypercholesterolemia. Report of the Program on the Surgical Control of the Hyperlipidemias (POSCH). *N Engl J Med* 1990; **323**: 946–55.

18. Buchwald H, Matts JP, Fitch LL, *et al*. For the POSCH Group. Changes in sequential coronary arteriograms and subsequent coronary events. *JAMA* 1992; **268**: 1429–33.

19. Steinberg D, Gotto AM. Preventing coronary artery disease by lowering cholesterol levels – fifty years from bench to bedside. *JAMA* 1999; **282**: 2043–50.

20. Libby P. Molecular basis of the acute coronary syndromes. *Circulation* 1995; **91**: 2844–50.

21. Steinberg D. Oxidative modification of LDL and atherogenesis. *Circulation* 1997; **95**: 1062–71.

22. Nickenig G, Harrison DG. The AT1-type receptor in oxidative stress and atherogenesis. Part I: oxidative stress and atherogenesis. *Circulation* 2002; **105**: 393–6.

23. Griendling KK, Sorescu D, Ushio-Fukai M. NAD(P)H oxidase: role in cardiovascular biology and disease. *Circ Res* 2000; **86**: 494–501.

24. Yusuf S, Dagenais G, Pogue J, *et al*. Vitamin E supplementation and cardiovascular events in high risk patients. The Heart Outcomes Prevention Evaluation Study Investigators. *N Engl J Med* 2000; **342**: 154–160.

25. GISSI-Prevenzione investigators. Dietary supplementation with n-3 polyunsaturated fatty acids and vitamin E after myocardial infarction: results of the GISSI-Prevenzione trial. Gruppo Italiano per lo Studio della Sopravvivenza nell infarto miocardio. *Lancet* 1999; **354**: 447–55.

26. Heart Protection Study Collaborative Group. MRC/BHF Heart Protection Study of Cholesterol Lowering with Simvastatin in 20 356 high-risk individuals: a randomised placebo-controlled trial. *Lancet* 2002; **360**: 7–22.

27. Chowienczyk PJ, Watts GF, Cockcroft JR, Ritter JM. Impaired endothelium-dependent vasodilation of forearm resistance vessels in hypercholesterolemia. *Lancet* 1992; **340**: 1430–2.

28. Vita JA, Yeung AC, Winniford M, *et al*. Effect of cholesterol lowering therapy on coronary endothelial vasomotor function in patients with coronary artery disease. *Circulation* 2000; **102**: 846–51.

29. Wilson SH, Simari RD, Best PJM, *et al*. Simvastatin preserves coronary endothelial function in hypercholesterolemia in the absence of lipid lowering. *Atheroscler Thromb Vasc Biol* 2001; **21**: 122–32.

30. Egashira K, Hirooka Y, Kai H, *et al*. Reduction in serum cholesterol with pravastatin improves endothelium-dependent coronary vasomotion in patients with hypercholesterolemia. *Circulation* 1994; **89**: 2519–24.

31. Treasure CB, Klein JL, Weintraub WS, *et al*. Beneficial effects of cholesterol-lowering therapy on the coronary endothelium in patients with coronary artery disease. *N Engl J Med* 1995; **332**: 481–7.

32. O'Driscoll G, Green D, Taylor RR. Simvastatin, an HMG-Coenzyme A reductase inhibitor, improves endothelial function within 1 month. *Circulation* 1997; **95**: 1126–31.

33. Dupuis J, Tardif JC, Cernacek P, Theroux P. Cholesterol reduction rapidly improves endothelial function after acute coronary syndromes. *Circulation* 1999; **99**: 3227–33.

34. Anderson T, Meredith IT, Yeung AC, Frei B, Selwyn AP, Ganz P. The effect of cholesterol-lowering and antioxidant therapy on endothelial-dependent coronary vasomotion. *N Engl J Med* 1995; **332**: 488–93.

35. Van Bowen AJ, Jukema JW, Zwinderman AH, *et al*. Reduction of transient myocardial ischemia with pravastatin in addition to the conventional treatment in patients with angina pectoris. *Circulation* 1996; **94**: 1503–5.

36. Andrews TC, Raby K, Barry J, *et al*. Effect of cholesterol reduction on myocardial ischemia in patients with coronary artery disease. *Circulation* 1997; **97**: 324–8.

37. Ross R. Atherosclerosis – an inflammatory disease. *N Engl J Med* 1999; **340**: 115–26.

38. Ridker PM, Rifai N, Clearfield M, *et al*. Measurement of c-reactive protein for the targeting of statin therapy in the primary prevention of acute coronary events. *N Engl J Med* 2001; **344**: 1959–65.

39. Ridker PM. On evolutionary biology, inflammation, infection, and the causes of atherosclerosis. *Circulation* 2002; **105**: 2–4.

40. Pitts B, Waters D, Brown WV, *et al*. Aggressive lipid-lowering therapy compared with angioplasty in stable coronary artery disease. *N Engl J Med* 1999; **341**: 70–6.

41. Schwartz GG, Olsson AN, Ezekowitz MD, *et al*. Effects of atorvastatin on early recurrent ischemic events in acute coronary syndromes – The MIRACL Study: a randomized controlled trial. *JAMA* 2001; **285**: 1711–18.

42. Walter D, Fichtlscherer S, Britten MB, *et al*. Benefits of immediate initiation of statin therapy following successful coronary stent implantation in patients with stable and unstable angina pectoris and Q-wave myocardial infarction. *Am J Cardiol* 2002; **89**: 1–6.

43. Azen SP, Mack WJ, Cashin-Hemphill L, *et al*. Progression of coronary artery disease predicts clinical coronary events: long-term follow-up from the Cholesterol Lowering Atherosclerosis Study. *Circulation* 1996; **93**: 34–41.

44. MAAS Investigators. Effect of simvastatin on coronary atheroma: The Multicenter Anti-Atheroma Study (MAAS). *Lancet* 1994; **344**: 633–8.

45. Crouse JR III, Byington RP, Bond MA, *et al*. Pravastatin, lipids and atherosclerosis in the carotid arteries (PLAC-II). *Am J Cardiol* 1995; **75**: 455–9.

46. Jukema JW, Bruschke AVG, Van Boven AJ, *et al*. Effects of lipid lowering by pravastatin an progression and regression of coronary artery disease in symptomatic men with normal to moderately elevated serum cholesterol levels. The Regression Growth Evaluation Statin Study (REGRESS). *Circulation* 1995; **91**: 2528–40.

47. Post Coronary Artery Graft Trial Investigators. The effect of aggressive lowering of low-

density lipoprotein cholesterol levels and low-dose anticoagulation on obstructive changes in saphenous vein coronary-artery bypass grafts. *N Engl J Med* 1997; **336**: 153–62.

48. Waters D, Higginson L, Gladstone P, *et al.* Effects of monotherapy with a reductase inhibitor on the progression of coronary atherosclerosis as assessed by serial quantitative arteriography. The Canadian Coronary Atherosclerosis Intervention Trial. *Circulation* 1994; **89**: 959–68.

49. Farmer JA. Pleiotropic effects of statins. *Curr Atheroscler Rep* 2000; **2**: 208–17.

50. Sparrow CP, Burton CA, Hernandez M, *et al.* Simvastatin has anti-inflammatory and anti-atherosclerotic activities independent of plasma cholesterol. *Arterioscler Thromb Vasc Biol* 2001; **21**: 115–21.

51. Laufs U, Fafata V, Plutzky J, Liao JK. Upregulation of endothelial nitric oxide synthase by HMG CoA reductase inhibitors. *Circulation* 1998; **97**: 1129–36.

52. Stenestrand U, Wallentin L. Early statin treatment following acute myocardial infarction and 1-year survival. *JAMA* 2001; **285**: 430–6.

53. Aronow HD, Topol EJ, Roe MT, *et al.* Effect of lipid-lowering therapy on early mortality after acute coronary syndromes: an observational study. *Lancet* 2001; **357**: 1063–8.

54. Brown GB, Zhao X-Q, Chait A, *et al.* Niacin plus simvastatin, but not antioxidant vitamins, protect against atherosclerosis and clinical events in CAD patients with low HDLC. *N Engl J Med* 2001; **345**: 1583–92.

Appendix Randomized clinical trials in dyslipidemia: important trials since 1994

SECONDARY PREVENTION TRIALS WITH STATINS: SIX TRIALS

Primary endpoint in all: CAD death plus non-fatal MI

Scandinavian Simvastatin Survival Study (4S)

Year: 1994
Population: Very high-risk. 4444 subjects with established CAD
Baseline lipids: TC 260, LDL 186, HDL 46, TG 141
Follow-up: 5.4 years

Results: Relative risk reduction (RR) of 34% in primary endpoint, p <0.00001
* Decrease in total and CAD deaths
* Decrease in revascularization
* Comparable results in diabetics, women, the elderly
* At 2-year post-study follow-up, the absolute survival advantage of statin-treated subjects widened, and the relative risk reduction remained at 30%, p = 0.0002

Lipid reduction: TC −25%, LDL −35%, HDL +8%
Placebo event rate: 5% per year
Drug: Simvastatin 20–40 mg or placebo
Citation: Lancet 1994; **344**: 1383–9; *Am J Cardiol* 2000; **86**: 257–62.

Cholesterol and recurrent events (CARE)

Year: 1996
Population: Moderate risk. 4159 post-MI subjects
Baseline lipids: TC 209, LDL 139, HDL 38, TG 156
Follow-up: 5 years

Results: RR reduction of 24% in primary endpoint, p = 0.003
* Decrease in revascularization
* Decrease in stroke

Lipid reduction: TC −20%, LDL −32%, HDL +5%, TG −14%

Placebo event rate: 2.7% per year (3.5% per year if aged over 65 years)
Drug: Pravastatin 40 mg or placebo
Citation: N Engl J Med 1996; **335**: 1001–9.

Long-term intervention with pravastatin in ischemic disease (LIPID)

Year: 1998
Population: Moderate risk. 9014 subjects with established CAD (prior MI in two-thirds)
Baseline lipids: TC 218, LDL 150, HDL 36, TG 140
Follow-up: 6 years

Results: RR reduction of 24% in primary endpoint, p = 0.0004
• Decrease in total mortality
• Decrease in revascularization
• Decrease in stroke
• Decrease CAD mortality of 31% in women with additional 2-year follow-up (non-randomized)

Lipid reduction: TC –18%, LDL –25%, HDL +6%, TG –12%
Placebo event rate: 2.6% per year
Drug: Pravastatin 40 mg/dL or placebo
Citation: N Engl J Med 1998; **339**: 1349–57; J Am Coll Cardiol 2001; **37** (Suppl. A): 262A.

PRIMARY PREVENTION TRIALS WITH STATINS: TWO TRIALS

Primary endpoint: CAD death plus non-fatal MI

Prevention of coronary heart disease with pravastatin in men with hypercholesterolemia (WOSCOPS or Western Scotland)

Year: 1995
Population: 6595 men, aged 45–64 years, high-risk subjects with very high TC and LDL
Baseline lipids: TC 272, LDL 192, HDL 44, TG 162
Follow-up: 4.9 years. Additional follow-up 3 years after study completion

Results: RR reduction of 31% in primary endpoint, p = 0.001
• Decrease total mortality
• Decrease revascularization
• At 3-year post-study follow-up, event curves and risk reduction for total and cardiovascular mortality unaltered in subjects who did not have a clinical event during the randomized study. Only 15% of these patients on lipid therapy

Lipid reduction: TC −20%, LDL −26%, HDL +5%, TG −12%
Placebo event rate: 1.6% per year
Drug: Pravastatin 40 mg
Citation: N Engl J Med 1995; **333**: 1301–7; J Am Coll Cardiol 2001; **37** (Suppl. A) 220A.

Air Force/Texas Coronary Atherosclerosis Prevention Study (AF CAPS/TEX CAPS)

Year: 1998
Population: 6505 low-risk subjects with low HDL and normal to mildly elevated LDL
Baseline lipids: TC 221, LDL 150, HDL 36, TG 158
Follow-up: 5.2 years

Results: RR reduction of 37% in first CAD event, including unstable angina, sudden death, fatal or non-fatal MI (p = 0. 001)
Note: Broader composite endpoint than in other trials
• Decrease in revascularization

Lipid reduction: TC −18%, LDL −25%, HDL +6%, TG −15% (at lipid levels year one of study)
Placebo event rate: 1.1% per year, including unstable angina; 0.7% per year (estimated) for CAD death and non-fatal MI alone, excluding unstable angina
Drug: Lovastatin 20–40 mg or placebo
Citation: JAMA 1998; **279**: 1615–22.

OTHER RECENT IMPORTANT LIPID LOWERING STUDIES: FIVE TRIALS

Post Coronary Artery Bypass Graft (CABG) trial

Year: 1997
Population: 1351 post-saphenous vein CABG (aged 1–11 years) patients with elevated LDL, preserved LV function, and at least one to two patent grafts
Baseline lipids: TC 225, LDL 155, HDL 38, TG 160
Follow-up: Serial angiograms at baseline and 4–5 years (4.3 years average). Additional follow-up 3 years after study completion
Regimen: 2 × 2 factorial design, two doses of lovastatin; low-dose coumadin, placebo; resin could be added to achieve LDL target

Results: Primary endpoint: less vein graft disease progression (RR reduction 31%, p = <0.001); fewer new lesions in aggressive LDL group (RR reduction 46–52%)
• Less revascularization in aggressive LDL cohort
• Decrease in clinical endpoints
• At late 7.5-year follow-up (off study medication), 42% less revascularization and 24% decrease in clinical endpoints in aggressive LDL group. No decrease in mortality

- Low-dose anticoagulation associated with decreased mortality (35%) and death or MI (31%) versus placebo at late follow-up, but not at 4.3 years (off study medication)

Lipid reduction:
Aggressive: TC –30%, LDL –40%, HDL +5%, TG 0
Moderate: TC –9%, LDL –15%, HDL +4%, TG +18%
Drug: Moderate LDL reduction, 2.5 to 5 mg lovastatin (plus resin if needed)
Aggressive LDL reduction, 40 to 80 mg lovastatin (plus resin if needed)
      Warfarin 1–4 mg to achieve INR <2.0, or placebo
Citation: N Engl J Med 1997; **336**: 153–62; Circulation 2000; **102**: 157–65.

High–density lipoprotein cholesterol Intervention Trial (VA-HIT)

Year: 1999
Population: 2531 high-risk males with CAD, mean age 64 years. Obese, diabetes (25%)
Baseline lipids: TC 175, LDL 111, HDL 32, TG 160
Follow-up: 5.1 years
Primary endpoint: Non-fatal MI or CAD death

Results: RR reduction of 22% in primary endpoint, p = 0.006
- Stroke = trend toward decrease (25%)
- TIA = 59% decrease, p = 0.001
- Carotid endarterectomy = 65% decrease, p = 0.001
- No difference in revascularization, unstable angina

Lipid reduction: TC –4%, LDL –4%, HDL +6%, TG –31%
Placebo event rate: 4.3% per year
Drug: Gemfibrozil 600 mg b.i.d., or placebo
Citation: N Engl J Med 1999; **341**: 410–18.

Aggressive lipid–lowering therapy compared with angioplasty in stable coronary disease (AVERT)

Year: 1999
Population: 341 patients with stable CAD (asymptomatic or Class I–II angina, normal LV function), one or two coronary lesions (>75%), recommended for PTCA (LDL >115 mg/dL; TG <500 mg/dL)
Baseline lipids: TC 223, LDL 147, HDL 42, TG 165
Follow-up: 18 months
Primary endpoint (at least one): CV death, stroke, CABG, PTCA, unstable angina hospitalization

Results: Atorvastatin (A) decreased ischemic events by 36% (p = 0.048, NS), predominately due to decreased revascularization, 13% versus 21% and hospitalization for angina (6.7% versus 14.1%). A increased time to first event (p = 0.03). PTCA cohort had greater improvement in angina

Lipid reduction: A decreased LDL to 77 mg/dL (46%) versus usual care LDL decrease of 18%, 119 mg/dL (p = 0.05). TC fell 31% versus −10%, HDL increased 8% versus 11%, and TG decreased 11% versus 10%
Event rate: 9% versus 14% per year (any event), estimated
Drug: Atorvastatin 80 mg versus usual care
Citation: *N Engl J Med* 1999; **341**: 70–6.

Myocardial Ischemia Reduction with Aggressive Cholesterol Lowering trial (MIRACL)

Year: 2000
Population: 3086 subjects hospitalized with an acute coronary syndrome: unstable angina or non-Q MI, TC <270 mg/dL. Enrollment 'window' or period was 24–96 h from admission
Baseline lipids: TC 208, LDL 124, HDL 46, TG 184
Follow-up: 16 weeks
Primary endpoint: Composite of time to death, non-fatal MI, arrest, worsening angina requiring hospitalization with objective ischemia

Results: Composite endpoint decrease of 16% (CI 0.70–1.00), p = 0.048
• Atorvastatin 14.8% versus placebo 17.4%
• Worsening angina: Atorvastatin decreased 26% (CI 0.57–0.94), p = 0.02
• No difference in other endpoints
• Stroke decreased in atorvastatin cohort, RR 0.50 (p = 0.045)

Lipid reduction: TC −27%, LDL −40%, HDL +4%, TG −16% with statin; LDL = 12%, TC increased 9% with placebo
Drug: Atorvastatin 80 mg versus placebo
Citation: *JAMA* 2001; **285**: 1711–18.

HDL Atherosclerosis Treatment Study (HATS)

Year: 2000
Population: 160 patients with CAD, elevated LDL (34 mg/dL with diabetes or impaired fasting glucose) and HDL <35 mg/dL
Treatment: Four groups

1. Niacin-simvastatin (N-S) or placebo
2. Vitamins E, C, beta-carotene, selenium or placebo
3. N-S plus vitamins
4. N-S placebo – placebo

Baseline lipids: TC 191, LDL 125, HDL 31, TG 213
Follow-up: 3 years
Primary endpoint:
1. Quantitative coronary angiographic average change in % stenosis of the nine most severe coronary lesions
2. Clinical: time to first major CAD event

Results:
- Niacin-statin prevented progression
- Clinical events decreased by 70%
- Vitamins = no effect, lowered APO-1 and HDL
- Subsequent analysis suggests that N-S increases in HDL-2, apo A-1 and HDL particle size were attenuated by the anti-oxidant cocktail

Drug: Niacin 2–4 g (mean 2.5 g) plus simvastatin 10–20 mg (mean 13 mg) or placebo

Citation: *Circulation* 2000; **102**: 506; *J Am Coll Cardiol* 2001; **37** (Suppl. A): 262A; *J Am Coll Cardiol* 2001; **37** (Suppl. A): 268A; *Arterioscler Thromb Vasc Biol* 2001; **21**: 1320.

Heart Protection Study (HPS)

Year: 2002
Population: Moderate risk. 20 536 adults with a wide variation in vascular risk, including 13 386 (65%) subjects with CAD; 1820 with cerebrovascular disease; 2701 with peripheral vascular disease; and 3982 with diabetes (some patients had more than one of these conditions)
Baseline lipids: TC 228, LDL 130, HDL 41, TG 81
Follow-up: 5 years
Results: Risk reduction of 27% in primary endpoint of fatal CAD plus non-fatal MI, p = 0.0001
All endpoints showed a 24% reduction in relative risk across a wide variety of diagnoses, age, sex, and LDL-C level, p = 0.0001
- Decrease in total mortality
- Decrease in CAD mortality
- Decrease in coronary revascularization procedures
- Decrease in ischemic stroke
- Decrease carotid and peripheral artery revascularization procedures

Lipid reduction: *TC 20%; LDL –29%; HDL +2.5%; TG –15%
Placebo event rate: 2.4% per year
Drug: Simvastatin 40 mg or placebo
Citation: *Lancet* 2002: **360**: 7–22; www.hpsinfo.org

*By study termination at 5 years, there was considerable dropout of subjects on simvastatin as well as statin drop-in rates on placebo. Thus, differences between baseline and achieved lipid levels on simvastatin were lower than anticipated.

2

Lipids and atherosclerosis

BRADFORD C BERK AND DANIEL A WUTHRICH

INTRODUCTION

Elevated serum cholesterol is a major risk factor for the development of coronary heart disease. The first epidemiological evidence for cholesterol as a risk factor for cardiovascular disease appeared in the Multiple Risk Factor Intervention Trial, which demonstrated an increase of 14 deaths yearly per 1000 men with serum cholesterol greater than 244 mg/dL.[1] During the twentieth century, myocardial infarction (MI) surpassed infectious diseases in Western societies as the primary cause of death.

Vascular lesions, which are the precursors to acute ischemic coronary syndromes, are ubiquitous in modern populations and have been found in autopsy studies even in the very young. For more than 20 years, convincing research data have been available linking a high-cholesterol diet to atherosclerotic disease.[2] During the late 1970s Gerrity and coworkers[3] demonstrated in an animal model that just weeks after initiation of a high-cholesterol diet, alterations and injury to the vascular endothelium and intima occur. Indeed, after only 12 weeks of a high-cholesterol diet, areas of endothelial injury begin developing foam cell lesions – one of the earliest events associated with the atherosclerotic process.

Now, after 20 years of vascular and lipid research, many of the pathological and molecular mechanisms of atherosclerosis are being described. It is now widely accepted that the oxidation of lipids – and in particular that of low-density lipoprotein (LDL) – is a key step in the atherogenic process. In this chapter, the molecular mechanisms leading to coronary atherosclerotic disease, as well as the rationale of using anti-oxidants as therapy to prevent oxidation of lipids and vascular wall components will be examined.

Currently, progress is being made toward an understanding of the molecular and pathological events that link hypercholesterolemia to the development of atherosclerotic disease. Atherosclerotic lesions are hypothesized to form as an inflammatory response to injury in the arterial wall. There is evidence that hyperlipidemia has a direct role in the initial injury process and in arterial leukocyte recruitment; these elements constitute the basis for the formation of foam cell lesions. This process is thought to occur through a series of events whereby hyperlipidemia increases arterial reactive oxygen species (ROS, which are O_2^-, $OH^.$ and H_2O_2) production. Other pathological processes implicated in atherosclerosis – such as hypertension and ischemia/reperfusion – have also been shown to increase vascular ROS. ROS in turn can directly damage vascular endothelium, consume nitric oxide (NO) and increase transcription of reduction–oxidation (redox)-sensitive genes. Expression of adhesion molecule genes such as vascular cell adhesion molecule-1 (VCAM-1), intracellular adhesion molecule-1 (ICAM-1) and E-selectin is hypothesized to be an important part of early atherosclerosis (Figure 2.1). VCAM-

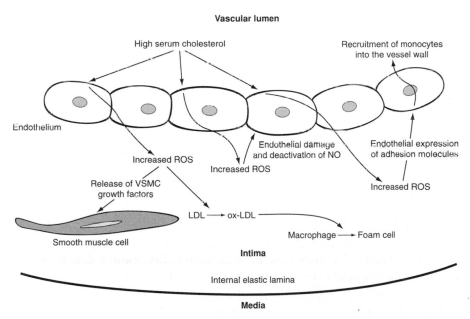

Figure 2.1 *A schemata showing oxidative stress-initiated events in the vascular wall. Although oxidation of LDL is very important in atherosclerosis, reactive oxygen species (ROS) are also thought to be important in a cascade of other events implicated in atherosclerotic disease. ROS can directly damage the vascular endothelium, consume nitric oxide and increase transcription of reduction-oxidation (redox)-sensitive genes, such as adhesion molecules. VSMC, vascular smooth muscle cell.*

1 is a molecular link that has redox-sensitive expression and has been shown to recruit inflammatory cells from the circulation into the arterial intima; indeed, VCAM-1 expression may be one of the earliest events leading to the formation of atherosclerosis.[4] Understanding the molecular and pathological events leading to the development of atherosclerosis provides insight into the treatment and prevention of heart disease.

ATHEROSCLEROSIS: ROS AND ENDOTHELIAL DYSFUNCTION

The energy of the oxygen molecule in living tissue is harvested when the molecule is reduced to water. In this enzymatically mediated process, oxygen accepts four electrons. ROS are formed when an oxygen molecule reduces O_2^-, OH and H_2O_2 by three or fewer electrons. The span of three ROS that can be formed if oxygen is incompletely reduced to water are: (i) superoxide anion radical, (O_2^-); (ii) hydroxyl radical (OH^-); and (iii) hydrogen peroxide (H_2O_2) (Figure 2.2). Sources of vascular free radicals are summarized in Box 2.1.

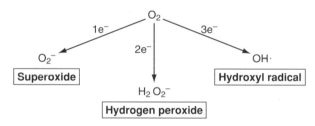

Figure 2.2 *The three reactive oxygen species (ROS) that can be formed if oxygen is incompletely reduced to water are: (i) superoxide anion radical; (ii) hydroxyl radical; and (iii) hydrogen peroxide.*

Box 2.1 *Sources of reactive oxygen species (ROS) in the vascular wall*

- Leakage from mitochondria
- Arachidonic acid metabolism by cyclooxygenase, cytochrome P-450 and lipoxygenase
- Xanthine metabolism by xanthine oxidase
- NADPH oxidases present in neutrophils and monocytes
- An NADH oxidase found in vascular smooth muscle cells which is structurally similar to the phagocytic NADPH

*Sources such as xanthine metabolism are important in ischemia reperfusion injury. Vascular NADH oxidase appears to be humorally regulated, and angiotensin II appears to play an important role in its induction

---

Mammalian tissues rely on the presence of antioxidants (e.g. glutathione and butyrate) and detoxifying enzymes (e.g. superoxide dismutase) to protect themselves from the ravages of ROS. ROS also interact with lipids and lipoproteins to cause their oxidation. There is now overwhelming evidence that oxidized lipoproteins are largely responsible for many of the pathological changes in the vascular wall associated with atherosclerosis. The various vascular effects hypothesized to occur secondary to ROS specifically through O_2^- and H_2O_2 are shown in Figure 2.3. Conversely, it has been shown that the administration of anti-oxidants can slow the progression of atherosclerosis in animal models.[6,7] Atherosclerosis has long been associated with abnormal vascular relaxation and tone, and much of this dysfunction can be attributed to aberrant function of the vascular endothelium.[8] Endothelial relaxation is mediated biologically by endothelial production and release of NO.[9] ROS are important in the regulation of vascular tone as NO can be rapidly consumed by superoxide anion and, conversely, NO is protected by superoxide dismutase – an enzyme which converts superoxide to a non-reactive species. In animal models, inhibition of NO production accelerates the development of atherosclerosis.[10]

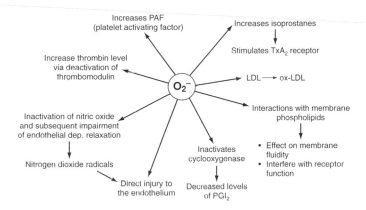

Figure 2.3 *The various vascular pro-atherogenic and pro-thrombotic effects hypothesized to occur secondary to reactive oxygen species (ROS), specifically through O_2^-, and H_2O_2. TxA, thromboxane; PGI, prostaglandin.*

There is evidence that hypercholesterolemia itself increases oxidant stress in vascular beds by increasing endothelial superoxide anion (O_2^-) production. Experiments carried out in hypercholesterolemic rabbits showed a three-fold increase in vascular superoxide production in those animals fed a high-cholesterol diet.[11] This increase was not observed if the vascular endothelium was removed,[11] and was not related to macrophage infiltration.[12] On an optimistic note, these studies also demonstrated that normalizing the dietary cholesterol for 1 month improved vascular relaxation and normalized vascular endothelial O_2^- production.[12]

Although in humans it is difficult to measure hypercholesterolemia-induced superoxide production in the vascular wall, such production can be inferred by studying vascular tone. In humans, the impaired vasodilation present in coronary atherosclerosis can be demonstrated by a paradoxical response to intracoronary infusion of acetylcholine (ACh): normal coronary arteries dilate in response to ACh infusion, while diseased arteries constrict.[13] This response is presumed to be the manifestation of redox changes in the vessel. In a study by Leung and coworkers,[14] 25 men with elevated serum cholesterol were treated with a low-fat diet and cholestyramine. Their response to ACh and nitroglycerin infusion was assessed by quantitative angiography at baseline, and after 6 months of therapy. These subjects, despite the normal angiographic appearance of their coronary arteries, had endothelial-mediated abnormal vascular tone (coronary vasoconstriction to ACh) prior to treatment. As in the rabbit models, impairment of endothelium-dependent dilation was found to be reversible. A subsequent study by Anderson and coworkers found that in patients treated with lipid-lowering agents, the vasodilator response to ACh is related to the susceptibility of LDL to oxidation. This suggests that oxidative stress itself is an important determinant of the coronary endothelial dysfunction observed in patients with atherosclerosis and hypercholesterolemia.[15]

In humans, improved endothelial function is inversely related to serum cholesterol concentrations after therapy. Overall in the Leung study, the patients went from a mean constrictive response prior to treatment to a normal coronary dilatation response after just 6 months of dietary and single-agent lipid therapy.[14] The results of these studies demonstrate that, in humans, endothelial dysfunction predates angiographic coronary abnormalities. In animal studies, the changes leading to endothelial dysfunction are hypothesized to be redox changes in the vessel wall. Furthermore, lesions not evident angiographically exhibit dysfunctional tone when NO – the endothelial-derived relaxation factor – is rapidly degraded by increased superoxide anion.

Although hypercholesterolemia has thus been identified as a cause of vascular endothelial dysfunction, other causes have been implicated more recently. Angiotensin II – which is a vasoactive peptide hormone and one of the most potent vasoconstrictors yet identified – may itself be a humoral factor implicated in endothelial dysfunction by altering production of ROS. Angiotensin-converting enzyme (ACE) catalyzes the final reaction in angiotensin II synthesis.

In the TREND (Trial on Reversing Endothelial Dysfunction) study, Mancini and coworkers[16] found that treatment with the ACE inhibitor quinapril had a substantial effect in improving endothelial dysfunction in normotensive patients with known coronary artery disease. This response was similar to the endothelial vasomotor improvement reported with lipid-lowering intervention. One of the proposed mechanisms for this effect involves angiotensin II modulation of vascular superoxide production; it has now been shown that angiotensin II can increase superoxide by inducing and activating vascular NADH oxidases present in vascular smooth muscle cells.[17]

In early 2000, the results of the HOPE (Heart Outcomes Prevention Evaluation) study were published, and these demonstrated a robust decrease in a variety of clinical endpoints in 9500 patients aged over 55 years who had established vascular disease or diabetes, and were treated with the ACE inhibitor ramipril for 4–5 years.[18] This important study suggests that older, high-risk subjects should be treated with an ACE inhibitor as part of standard therapy for prevention of vascular morbidity and mortality.

In summary, there is good evidence that a high serum cholesterol level can directly alter the redox state in the vessel wall and initiate the cascade of events associated with early atherosclerosis and vascular dysfunction. Increased superoxide production has myriad effects, including the destruction of NO, increased lipid oxidation, changes in gene expression, and post-translational activation and deactivation of proteins. One of the more important events is the oxidation and modification of LDL. The oxidized form of LDL is preferentially taken up by the scavenger receptor of the macrophages to form foam cells. Oxidized LDL is itself injurious to cells, and may directly cause a reactive inflammatory response in the arterial wall. Hypercholesterolemia is not the only 'injury' to cause vascular endothelial dysfunction; angiotensin II may have a similar and additive effect, causing changes in vascular redox state.[19] Evidence has now been obtained from human angiographic trials that either lowering serum cholesterol or inhibiting angiotensin II synthesis results in improved endothelial vasomotor function in patients with coronary atherosclerotic disease.

LDL AND VASCULAR REDOX STATE EFFECTS ON VASCULAR PHENOTYPE

For the long-term progression of atherosclerosis, one would hypothesize the occurrence of phenotypic changes in the endothelium and vascular smooth muscle cells. These phenotypic changes can result from at least two different mechanisms: (i) post-translational modification of pre-existing proteins; and/or (ii) changes in gene expression (transcriptional regulation).

Ample data exist which show that oxidized LDL has multiple effects on transcriptional and post-transcriptional regulatory factors. Early atherosclerotic lesions in humans as well as animals have been shown to have accumulation of oxidized lipoproteins. The presence of oxidized LDL can have important effects on gene expression. For instance, platelet-derived growth factor (PDGF) is produced and secreted by many of the cell types that take part in the atherogenic process and it is oxidized LDL – not native LDL – that stimulates expression of PDGF-B and its secretion in macrophages.[20] Another mechanism by which the inflammatory response of the early atherosclerotic lesion could be initiated and sustained is by endothelial cell expression of factors that attract immune cells and stimulate their proliferation. Lipid peroxidation and redox state have now been shown to be important factors in regulating the adhesion molecule VCAM-1.[21] Moreover, Rajavashisth and coworkers have shown recently that the exposure of oxidized LDL to cultured endothelial cells results in a large and rapid increase in the expression of multiple macrophage and granulocyte chemotactic factors and growth factors.[22] One of the more important genes induced by oxidized LDL is the monocyte-chemotactic protein-1 (MCP-1), which may have important effects in attracting macrophages to a newly forming atherosclerotic lesion.

It is hypothesized that these types of phenotypic changes would occur through redox-sensitive transcriptional or post-transcriptional regulatory factors. In early atherosclerosis, adhesion molecules expressed on the surface of vascular endothelial cells selectively recruit monocytes into the newly forming lesions. VCAM-1 has been shown to have such a role.[23] Physically, VCAM-1 is an immunoglobulin receptor, which is expressed on the endothelial cell surface. Receptors and ligands interact in a manner analogous to a 'lock and key,' where the receptor is the 'lock' and the receptor's ligand is the matching 'key.' Only specific immune cells have ligands that match the VCAM-1 receptor. One of the VCAM-1 ligands has been shown to be very late activation antigen-4 (VLA-4), which is expressed on monocytes and lymphocytes.[24] Thus, when circulating monocytes contact vascular endothelium that has VCAM-1 expressed on their cell surface, the 'lock and key' join together and the immune cells are physically recruited to the lesion area. After binding to VCAM-1, monocytes migrate between the endothelial cells and localize sub-endothelially. Once monocytes leave the circulation they are termed macrophages. The recruited macrophages can then become foam cells as their scavenger receptors take up oxidized LDL and they become lipid-laden.

More recently, gene transcription and expression of VCAM-1 have been shown to be regulated by a redox-sensitive mechanism in human endothelial cells.[4] In this study, an anti-oxidant was able to block VCAM-1-mediated cell adhesion, as well as decrease VCAM-1 protein and mRNA levels. Since VCAM-1 gene expression is altered by the redox state, either it – or expression of a similar receptor – could be one of the earliest molecular events in atherosclerosis.

The mechanism by which vascular redox state regulates gene expression is not yet clearly understood, but it appears that redox-sensitive transcriptional factors such as nuclear factor kB (NF-kB) may play a role.[4,25] More recently, it has been shown that NO itself may function as an important modulator of redox-sensitive gene expression in the vasculature.[21]

HIGH-DENSITY LIPOPROTEIN (HDL) CHOLESTEROL

There is an inverse relationship between serum concentrations of HDL and coronary heart disease. There are at least two mechanisms responsible for this phenomenon. First, reverse-cholesterol transport HDL is largely responsible for removing arterial lipids and transporting them back to the liver; thus, high serum HDL levels represent a robust arterial system for removing atherogenic lipids from the vascular wall. Second, there is evidence that HDL itself – as well as HDL-associated enzymes – play a role in the prevention of LDL oxidation.

There are several proposed mechanisms by which HDL may provide this protective anti-oxidant effect. HDL has been shown *in vitro* to be a scavenger of superoxide, which indicates that it may have direct anti-oxidant action. There is also mounting evidence that HDL possesses a mechanism to abolish the activity of lysophosphatidylcholine (lyso-PC), which would indirectly protect LDL against lipid peroxidation. In addition, enzymes associated with HDL such as paraoxonase, acyltransferases and others may play a role in preventing LDL oxidation.[26]

HDL is a difficult risk factor to modify in patients. Most pharmacological interventions have only a small impact on HDL serum concentration, and some cholesterol-reducing agents can actually decrease HDL. One of the best strategies for increasing HDL is frequent aerobic exercise. Niacin, by unknown mechanisms, can also significantly increase HDL levels. Recently, in the VA-HIT trial, gemfibrizol was shown to be effective in preventing cardiovascular events; this study of males with established coronary disease, low HDL and normal LDL cholesterol, demonstrated a 22 percent reduction in a variety of cardiovascular endpoints with an average long-term therapy and follow-up of 5.1 years.[27]

EFFECT OF LIPID-LOWERING INTERVENTIONS

Although the association of high serum lipids with coronary artery disease has been known for some time, only very recently have trials shown that lipid-lowering therapy can prolong life. Five important recent studies involved a class of drugs that inhibit hydroxyl-methylglutaryl coenzyme A (HMG-CoA) reductase (see Chapter 1). These drugs – pravastatin, atorvostatin and simvastatin – are members of a class of drugs collectively referred to as the 'statins' or, alternatively, as HMG-CoA reductase inhibitors. These inhibitors block the enzyme responsible for the rate-limiting reaction in hepatic cholesterol synthesis, and this results in significant reductions of the serum levels of total and LDL cholesterol. Although numerous previous studies showed that drug therapy for hypercholesterolemia could significantly reduce the incidence of coronary events such as MI and angina, the effect of these pharmacological agents on mortality was less clear. In the first two statin studies, the Scandinavian Simvastatin Survival Study (4S)[28] and the West of Scotland Study,[29] pharmacological lipid-lowering therapy had dramatic effect. The 4S study was the first to demonstrate prolongation of life in secondary prevention–treatment of people with already diagnosed cardiovascular disease.[28] The West of Scotland Study demonstrated a decreased death rate in men from cardiovascular causes in primary prevention–treatment of people with no known cardiovascular disease.[29] Most recently, the GREACE study showed a significant decrease in mortality in a secondary prevention trial with atorvastatin versus usual care.[30] All three of these landmark controlled trials demonstrated the profound effect that the lowering of LDL cholesterol has on cardiovascular disease.

The Scandinavian Simvastatin Survival Study (4S) Group enrolled 4444 patients with angina or with previous MI and elevated serum cholesterol. The study was double-blind and placebo-controlled in nature. After approximately 5 years of follow-up, total cholesterol and LDL cholesterol had been reduced 25 percent and 35 percent respectively in the simvastatin-treated patients. Overall mortality was decreased by 30 percent ($p = 0.0003$), and mortality due to cardiovascular causes decreased significantly, by 42 percent. Major coronary events decreased significantly and approximately equally in both men and women (34 and 35%, respectively).

The West of Scotland Coronary Prevention Study is considered a primary prevention trial, although it is not purely such because 5 percent of patients enrolled had a history of stable angina. None, however, had a history of MI and all had a normal baseline ECG. This trial assigned 6595 middle-aged men with elevated cholesterol to receive either pravastatin or placebo. After an approximately 5-year mean follow-up, total cholesterol and LDL cholesterol had been reduced 20 percent and 36 percent, respectively. In the pravastatin-treated patients, overall mortality was decreased by 22 percent, which was almost significant ($p = 0.051$). Cardiovascular-related mortality decreased significantly, by 32 percent ($p = 0.033$). Major coronary events were decreased by 31 percent (p <0.001), and the combined endpoint of non-fatal MI or death was significantly reduced by 31 percent (p <0.001). The fact that this study did not include women and studied almost exclusively middle-aged white males with a high proportion of current smokers (44%) somewhat limits its applicability to diverse patient populations. Other statin trials – CARE, LIPID, and AFCAPS-TEXCAPS – have shown similar results in a variety of populations with differing lipid levels (see Chapter 1).

The recent Greek Atorvastatin and Coronary-heart-disease Evaluation (GREACE) Study[30] compared a structured lipid lowering treatment versus usual care in 1600 patients with coronary heart disease. The structured care arm sought to achieve an LDL of less than or equal to 100 mg/dL with atorvastatin. With atorvostatin and structured care, this study demonstrated not only a significant decrease in coronary events but also a significant decrease in overall mortality.[30]

THE ROLE OF ANTI-OXIDANTS IN THE PREVENTION OF ATHEROSCLEROSIS

Earlier in this chapter the roles of oxidized LDL and ROS in the atherogenic process were discussed in detail. Hyperlipidemia has been shown to increase arterial ROS production. These ROS can cause alterations and oxidation of lipids as well as directly damage the vascular endothelium. Since oxidized LDL is more atherogenic than non-oxidized LDL, and endothelial injury is presumed to be an initiating event in atherosclerotic formation, then inhibition of ROS with anti-oxidants could inhibit the progression of atherosclerosis. Dietary anti-oxidants may work together with HDL to scavenge superoxide and other ROS and thus protect LDL from pro-atherogenic oxidation. Anti-oxidants also inhibit other deleterious events such as direct endothelial damage and dysfunction by ROS. In experimental models, anti-oxidants have been shown to inhibit the adhesion of white cells to the vascular wall and also to inhibit platelet aggregation – all of which are important events in coronary disease and acute myocardial infarction.

Several antioxidants including vitamin C, vitamin E, probucol, and β-carotene have been studied for their effect on the progression of atherosclerotic vascular disease. Vitamin C has some theoretical advantages over the other anti-oxidants as it is active in the aqueous phase. In animal models, some of the initiating events of atherosclerosis – such as oxidized LDL-induced leukocyte adhesion to arterial endothelium and platelet aggregation – were completely prevented by vitamin C, but not by vitamin E or probucol.[31]

A small study of restenosis based on exercise thallium testing showed a benefit of vitamin E to limit restenosis.[32] In a secondary prevention trial – the Cambridge Heart Anti-oxidant Study (CHAOS) – dietary supplementation with high-dose vitamin E demonstrated significant cardiovascular benefit. CHAOS was randomized, double-blinded and placebo-controlled in nature. High-dose vitamin E (400 or 800 IU) was studied in 2002 patients with angiographically proven atherosclerotic disease and, after 200 days, a vitamin E treatment effect became apparent. At the end of the study, which had a median duration of follow-up of approximately 1.5 years, a dramatic benefit was seen in the vitamin E group with a 77 percent (p <0.001) decrease in the incidence of non-fatal MI. The combined endpoint of cardiovascular death or non-fatal MI was also significantly reduced by 47 percent (p <0.005). Among the vitamin E-treated patients, overall mortality was insignificantly increased (3.5% versus 2.7%, p = 0.31). Mortality due to cardiovascular problems was similar in both treated and untreated patients (2.6% versus 2.4% respectively; p = 0.78). Major coronary events, however, were significantly decreased, by 31 percent (p <0.001). This paradox could be explained if vitamin E had a greater effect in preventing non-fatal rather than fatal MI. This divergence of effect was also seen in the recently published α-tocopherol, β-carotene prevention study (ATBC)[33] in which low-dose vitamin E significantly decreased non-fatal MI (risk reduction of 38%), though – like CHAOS – no significant effect was seen on fatal events.

Vitamin E also showed benefit in the Cholesterol Lowering Atherosclerosis Study (CLAS). The results of ultrasound quantification of the distal common carotid artery showed that supplementary vitamin E intake reduced atherosclerotic progression in a subset of patients studied. In CLAS, vitamin C had no effect on carotid atherosclerotic progression in any group.[34] Vitamin E supplementation in epidemiological studies has been associated with a reduced incidence of MI and cardiovascular death in both men and women.[35,36] Although vitamin E has been believed to be the most promising anti-oxidant for the prevention of atherosclerosis, newer data do not support this; primary prevention studies with low doses of vitamin E have shown no significant benefit. Two recent large clinical trials have failed to show any benefit from vitamin E, however. Quite disappointingly – higher dose vitamin E in the secondary prevention HOPE trial had no effect on mortality or cardiac events. In the vitamin E arm there was no apparent benefit for a variety of vascular disease endpoints in over 9000 older subjects with established coronary, peripheral, or cerebrovascular disease, or in diabetics with one other coronary risk factor.[18] Also in GISSI-P, a post-MI trial of Italian subjects, vitamin E failed to produce any clinical benefits.[37] Thus, vitamin E as a single agent antioxidant is no longer considered a promising therapy for cardiovascular disease.[18] The combination of vitamin C and E could potentially be more effective than either vitamin alone because in biological systems vitamin C can 'regenerate' oxidized vitamin E, though this combination has not been tested in large-scale clinical trials.

To date, probucol and β-carotene appear to be even less promising anti-oxidants for the prevention of coronary artery disease. In the ATBC study there was a higher incidence of lung cancer and an increased mortality from ischemic heart disease in smokers receiving β-carotene.[38] In the Probucol Quantitative Regression Swedish Trial (PQRST), probucol appeared to protect against LDL oxidation in hypercholesterolemic patients with established atherosclerosis. This protection, however, was not found to alter progression or regression of femoral atherosclerosis significantly as assessed by quantitative arteriography.[39] The lack of efficacy of probucol may be due to the fact that it reduces serum HDL levels, which may offset the beneficial anti-oxidant effect. However, three studies have shown a beneficial effect of probucol on restenosis after angioplasty,[40–42] and the results of one study were negative.[40] Lee et al., in the PART study, found a significant decrease in restenosis among patients who received probucol, but this benefit was observed only in those patients who received 30 days of pretreatment.[42] Watanabe et al. found a similar benefit of probucol when administered 7 days prior to percutaneous transluminal coronary angioplasty (PTCA).[41] Tardif *et al.*, in the MVP study, compared probucol and multivitamins (β-carotene, vitamin E, and vitamin C) alone or in combination with 28 days of pretreatment. These authors found a significant decrease in restenosis with probucol, but not with the multivitamins.[39] Finally, O'Keefe *et al.* in the APPLE study found no benefit of lovastatin and probucol together on either clinical events, exercise thallium, or angiographic restenosis.[43] It should be noted that probucol was given 2 days before to 1 day after PTCA in this last study. The MVP study is the only study to compare anti-oxidant vitamins with probucol directly. This study was well designed in that treatment was initiated 28 days prior to angioplasty. The reasons why anti-oxidant vitamins failed to limit restenosis in the MVP study are not clear, but concomitant treatment with β-carotene may have exerted a harmful effect. Alternatively, longer follow-up may be required to observe any beneficial effects of anti-oxidant vitamins, as suggested by the CHAOS trial where differences with vitamin E were not observed for more than one year.[44]

In summary, the only anti-oxidants to show limited benefit in small human trials are vitamin E and probucol. In large secondary prevention trials vitamin E did not show benefit. While probucol showed apparent benefit in restenosis, its use in prevention of atherosclerosis is unwarranted at this time, especially since probucol lowers HDL. This drug is no longer available in the United States. Given the conflicting data on the role of vitamin E in secondary prevention of CAD, and the recent results of large-scale randomized trials there is currently no role for anti-oxidants in the treatment of cardiovascular disease. Moreover, there are currently no convincing data available of mortality benefit, and so their routine use in the treatment or prevention of coronary artery disease is not indicated at the present time.

A SUMMARY OF LIPID-LOWERING THERAPY

Over the past two decades, our understanding of ischemic heart disease – through basic science, epidemiology, and controlled trials – has greatly increased. How does all this knowledge translate into therapeutic recommendations? Certainly, the accumulated evidence supports a concept that a heart-healthy diet and exercise should be encouraged in all individuals. Cholesterol levels can be lowered by approximately 10 percent with aggressive dietary intervention, and exercise is one of the few ways known to increase serum levels of HDL, both of which have been shown epidemiologically to decrease cardiovascular events.

Screening of men and women over the age of 30 years for hypercholesterolemia should be carried out routinely. An elevated serum cholesterol that is unresponsive to diet should be treated with statins (based on NCEP guidelines), and if low HDL is present (<35 mg/dL) the addition of niacin should be considered.

Individuals with known coronary artery disease, or with more than two risk factors for developing coronary artery disease, might consider high-dose vitamin E regardless of their cholesterol status in order to prevent the pro-atherogenic effects of lipid oxidation, although the available data for such an approach are disappointing. The role of other anti-oxidants is unclear: vitamin C works well with vitamin E to further prevent oxidation and is quite effective in animal models; thus, even in the absence of clinical data it may be reasonable to recommend these two anti-oxidants together in high-risk individuals. Recently acquired data on β-carotene are of particular concern, and use of this anti-oxidant in the prevention of coronary artery disease should be discouraged, especially as some studies have shown a significant increase in cardiovascular events with its use. The ongoing clinical trials discussed earlier should further delineate the role of anti-oxidants in the primary and secondary treatment of cardiovascular disease.

It should be emphasized that in individuals with known heart disease, pharmacological cholesterol lowering with statins saves lives. Cholesterol levels should be monitored 6 weeks after a change in medication in order to insure an adequate treatment effect. The target LDL in patients with documented vascular disease is <100 mg/dL. Double and triple therapy with the addition of niacin or a fibrate, or bile acid-binding resins, should be utilized to normalize cholesterol concentrations in those people with known heart disease. Approaches to lipid-lowering therapy are discussed in detail in Chapters 6, 8 and 10.

SUMMARY

Hypercholesterolemia is a major risk factor for the development of coronary atherosclerotic disease. We now understand some of the mechanisms by which high serum cholesterol can lead directly to vascular injury. Many of the early events of plaque formation are coupled to redox changes in the vessel wall. Increased ROS production – which in animal models can be caused solely by a high-cholesterol diet – may be the initiating factor in vascular dysfunctional tone and relaxation. Furthermore, oxidation of LDL and redox-sensitive changes in gene expression may contribute to a series of events leading to localized inflammation and lesion progression. A summary of the postulated vascular events is shown in Figure 2.4. HDL, which traditionally is viewed as being important only in the context of reverse cholesterol transport, is now seen as an anti-oxidant with associated enzymes that protect LDL from oxidation.

Pharmacological treatment to lower cholesterol has now been shown to be effective in decreasing coronary events and, in some instances, prolonging life. The most dramatically effective treatment thus far has been with lipid-lowering therapy utilizing HMG-CoA reductase inhibitors to reduce both LDL and total cholesterol. Divergent humoral and systemic factors are now thought to contribute to the progression of atherosclerosis through the common pathway of increasing vascular ROS. Novel treatments of atherosclerosis using anti-oxidants or ACE inhibitors appear to have great potential, but this needs to be further evaluated in large-scale trials. Future therapies to block the genetic expression of genes involved in the initiating events of atherosclerotic lesions are currently being studied in animal models of atherosclerosis.

In this chapter the main focus has been on the role of cholesterol and lipids on the pathogenesis of atherosclerosis. However, high serum cholesterol is only one possible

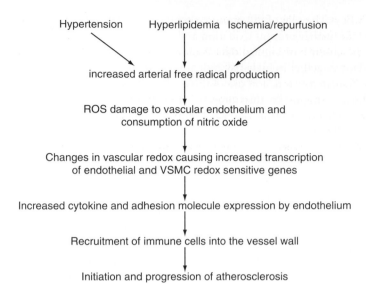

Figure 2.4 *Other pathological processes implicated in atherosclerosis, such as hypertension and ischemia/reperfusion have also been shown to increase vascular reactive oxygen species (ROS). As shown in the above diagram, ROS leads to a common sequence of events that can initiate and cause progression of atherosclerosis. VSMC, vascular smooth muscle cell.*

cause of vascular injury, and other factors act either in parallel or synergistically. Hypertension, genetic predisposition, diabetes, and tobacco use are major etiological agents in atherosclerotic initiation and progression. Furthermore T-cell-mediated immune responses, elevated homocysteine levels and infectious causes of atherosclerosis such as *Chlamydia* and cytomegalovirus are currently under investigation.

Studies in both animals and humans have shown that many of the initial pathological changes seen in hypercholesterolemia – especially those involving the vascular endothelium – are reversible if serum cholesterol levels are normalized. Angiographic studies in humans have also shown that lowering cholesterol can result in stabilization and in some cases overall regression of plaque burden in the coronary arteries. Moreover endothelial dysfunction, which is probably a causal factor in atherosclerotic lesion formation and progression, is also reversible with both lipid-lowering therapy and ACE inhibition. Further study of the molecular mechanisms of hypercholesterolemia-induced atherosclerosis will yield new insights into the treatment and prevention of acute coronary syndromes.

REFERENCES

1. Kannel WB, Neaton JD, Wentworth D, Thomas HE, Stamler J, Hulley SB, Kjelsberg MO. Overall and coronary heart disease mortality rates in relation to major risk factors in 325,348 men screened for the MRFIT. Multiple Risk Factor Intervention Trial. *Am Heart J* 1986; **112**: 825–36.

2. Ross R, Glomset JA. The pathogenesis of atherosclerosis (first of two parts). *N Engl J Med* 1976; **295**: 369–77.
3. Gerrity RG, Naito HK, Richardson M, Schwartz CJ. Dietary induced atherogenesis in swine. Morphology of the intima in prelesion stages. *Am J Pathol* 1979; **95**: 775–92.
4. Marui N, Offermann MK, Swerlick R, Kunsch C, Rosen CA, Ahmad M, Alexander RW, Medford RM. Vascular cell adhesion molecule-1 (VCAM-1) gene transcription and expression are regulated through an antioxidant-sensitive mechanism in human vascular endothelial cells. *J Clin Invest* 1993; **92**: 1866–74.
5. Crawford DW, Blakenhorn DH. Arterial wall oxygenation, oxyradicals, and atherosclerosis. *Atherosclerosis* 1991; **89**: 97–108.
6. Carew TE, Schwenke DC, Steinberg D. Antiatherogenic effect of probucol unrelated to its hypocholesterolemic effect: evidence that antioxidants in vivo can selectively inhibit low density lipoprotein degradation in macrophage-rich fatty streaks and slow the progression of atherosclerosis in the Watanabe heritable hyperlipidemic rabbit. *Proc Natl Acad Sci USA* 1987; **84**: 7725–9.
7. Kita T, Nagano Y, Yokode M, Ishii K, Kume N, Ooshima A, Yoshida H, Kawai C. Probucol prevents the progression of atherosclerosis in Watanabe heritable hyperlipidemic rabbit, an animal model for familial hypercholesterolemia. *Proc Natl Acad Sci USA* 1987; **84**: 5928–31.
8. Freiman PC, Mitchell GG, Heistad DD, Armstrong ML, Harrison DG. Atherosclerosis impairs endothelium-dependent vascular relaxation to acetylcholine and thrombin in primates. *Circ Res* 1986; **58**: 783–9.
9. Palmer R, Ferrige A, Moncada S. Nitric oxide release accounts for the biologic activity of endothelium-derived relaxing factor. *Nature* 1987; **327**: 524–6.
10. Cohen RA, Zitnay KM, Haudenschild CC, Cunningham LD. Loss of selective endothelial cell vasoactive functions caused by hypercholesterolemia in pig coronary arteries. *Circ Res* 1988; **63**: 903–10.
11. Ohara Y, Peterson TE, Harrison DG. Hypercholesterolemia increases endothelial superoxide anion production. *J Clin Invest* 1993; **91**: 2546–51.
12. Ohara Y, Peterson TE, Sayegh HS, Subramanian RR, Wilcox JN, Harrison DG. Dietary correction of hypercholesterolemia in the rabbit normalizes endothelial superoxide anion production. *Circulation* 1995; **92**: 898–903.
13. Ludmer PL, Selwyn AP, Shook TL, Wayne RR, Mudge GH, Alexander RW, Ganz P. Paradoxical vasoconstriction induced by acetylcholine in atherosclerotic coronary arteries. *N Engl J Med* 1986; **315**: 1046–51.
14. Leung WH, Lau CP, Wong CK. Beneficial effect of cholesterol-lowering therapy on coronary endothelium-dependent relaxation in hypercholesterolaemic patients. *Lancet* 1993; **341**: 1496–500.
15. Anderson TJ, Meredith IT, Charbonneau F, Yeung AC, Frei B, Selwyn AP, Ganz P. Endothelium-dependent coronary vasomotion relates to the susceptibility of LDL to oxidation in humans. *Circulation* 1996; **93**(9): 1647–50.
16. Mancini GB, Henry GC, Macaya C, O'Neill BJ, Pucillo AL, Carere RG, Wargovich TJ, Mudra H, Luscher TF, Klibaner MI, Haber HE, Uprichard AC, Pepine CJ, Pitt B. Angiotensin-converting enzyme inhibition with quinapril improves endothelial vasomotor dysfunction in patients with coronary artery disease. The TREND (Trial on Reversing ENdothelial Dysfunction) Study [see comments]. *Circulation* 1996; **94**: 258–65.
17. Griendling KK, Minieri CA, Ollerenshaw JD, Alexander RW. Angiotensin II stimulates NADH and NADPH oxidase activation in cultured vascular smooth muscle cells. *Circ Res* 1994; **74**: 1141–8.

18. Yusuf S, Sleight P, Pogue J, Bosch J, Davies R, Dagenais G. Effects of an angiotensin-converting-enzyme inhibitor, ramipril, on cardiovascular events in high-risk patients. The Heart Outcomes Prevention Evaluation Study Investigators. *N Engl J Med* 2000; **342**: 145–53.
19. Rajagopalan S, Kurz S, Munzel T, Tarpey M, Freeman BA, Griendling KK, Harrison DG. Angiotensin II-mediated hypertension in the rat increases vascular superoxide production via membrane NADH/NADPH oxidase activation. Contribution to alterations of vasomotor tone. *J Clin Invest* 1996; **97**: 1916–23.
20. Malden LT, Chait A, Raines EW, Ross R. The influence of oxidatively modified low density lipoproteins on expression of platelet-derived growth factor by human monocyte-derived macrophages. *J Biol Chem* 1991; **266**: 13901–7.
21. Khan BV, Harrison DG, Olbrych MT, Alexander RW, Medford RM. Nitric oxide regulates vascular cell adhesion molecule 1 gene expression and redox-sensitive transcriptional events in human vascular endothelial cells. *Proc Natl Acad Sci USA* 1996; **93**: 9114–19.
22. Rajavashisth TB, Andalibi A, Territo MC, Berliner JA, Navab M, Fogelman AM, Lusis AJ. Induction of endothelial cell expression of granulocyte and macrophage colony-stimulating factors by modified low-density lipoproteins. *Nature* 1990; **344**: 254–7.
23. Cybulsky MI, Gimbrone MA, Jr. Endothelial expression of a mononuclear leukocyte adhesion molecule during atherogenesis. *Science* 1991; **251**: 788–91.
24. Elices MJ, Osborn L, Takada Y, Crouse C, Luhowskyj S, Hemler ME, Lobb RR. VCAM-1 on activated endothelium interacts with the leukocyte integrin VLA-4 at a site distinct from the VLA-4/fibronectin binding site. *Cell* 1990; **60**: 577–84.
25. Schreck R, Meier B, Mannel DN, Droge W, Baeuerle PA. Dithiocarbamates as potent inhibitors of nuclear factor kappa B activation in intact cells. *J Exp Med* 1992; **175**: 1181–94.
26. Mackness MI, Durrington PN. HDL, its enzymes and its potential to influence lipid peroxidation. *Atherosclerosis* 1995; **115**: 243–53.
27. Rubins BH, Robbins SJ, Collins D, *et al*. Gemfibrozil for the secondary prevention of coronary heart disease in men with low levels of high-density lipoprotein cholesterol. *N Engl J Med* 1999; **341**: 410–18.
28. Group SSSS. Randomised trial of cholesterol lowering in 4444 patients with coronary heart disease: The Scandinavian Simvastatin Survival Study (4S). *Lancet* 1994; **344**: 1383–9.
29. Shepherd J, Cobbe SM, Ford I, Isles CG, Lorimer AR, MacFarlane PW, McKillop JH, Packard CJ. Prevention of coronary heart disease with pravastatin in men with hypercholesterolemia. West of Scotland Coronary Prevention Study Group. *N Engl J Med* 1995; **333**: 1301–7.
30. Athyros VG, Mikhailidis DP, Papageorgiou AA, Mercouris BR, Athyrou VV, Symeonidis AN, Basayannis EO, Demitriadis DS, Kontopoulos AG. Attaining United Kingdom-European Atherosclerosis Society low-density lipoprotein cholesterol guideline target values in the Greek Atorvastatin and Coronary-heart-disease Evaluation (GREACE) Study. *Curr Med Res Opin* 2002; **18(8)**: 499–502.
31. Lehr HA, Frei B, Olofsson AM, Carew TE, Arfors KE. Protection from oxidized LDL-induced leukocyte adhesion to microvascular and macrovascular endothelium in vivo by vitamin C but not by vitamin E. *Circulation* 1995; **91**: 1525–32.
32. Rimm EB, Stampfer MJ, Ascherio A, Giovannucci E, Colditz GA, Willett WC. Vitamin E consumption and the risk of coronary heart disease in men. *N Engl J Med* 1993; **328**: 1450–6.
33. Stampfer MJ, Hennekens CH, Manson JE, Colditz GA, Rosner B, Willett WC. Vitamin E consumption and the risk of coronary disease in women. *N Engl J Med* 1993; **328**: 1444–9.

34. DeMaio SJ, King SBI, Lembo NJ, Roubin GS, Hearn JA, Bhagavan HN, Sgoutas DS. Vitamin E supplementation, plasma lipids and incidence of restenosis after percutaneous transluminal coronary angioplasty (PTCA). *J Am Coll Nutr* 1992; **11**: 68–73.

35. The Alpha-Tocopherol BCCPSG. The effect of vitamin E and beta carotene on the incidence of lung cancer and other cancers in male smokers. *N Engl J Med* 1994; **330**: 1029–35.

36. Azen SP, Qian D, Mack WJ, Sevanian A, Selzer RH, Liu CR, Liu CH, Hodis HN. Effect of supplementary antioxidant vitamin intake on carotid arterial wall intima-media thickness in a controlled clinical trial of cholesterol lowering. *Circulation* 1996; **94**: 2369–72.

37. Gruppo Italiano per lo Studio della Sopravvivenza nell'Infarto miocardico. Dietary supplementation with n-3 polyunsaturated fatty acids and vitamin E after myocardial infarction: results of the GISSI-Prevenzione trial. Gruppo Italiano per lo Studio della Sopravvivenza nell'Infarto miocardico. *Lancet* 2001; **357**: 642.

38. Regnstrom J, Walldius G, Nilsson S, Elinder LS, Johansson J, Molgaard J, Holme I, Olsson AG, Nilsson J. The effect of probucol on low density lipoprotein oxidation and femoral atherosclerosis. *Atherosclerosis* 1996; **125**: 217–29.

39. Tardif J-C, Cote G, Lesperance J, Bourassa M, Bilodeau M, Doucet S, Tanguay J-F, deGuise P, Dupont C. Prevention of restenosis by pre and post-PTCA probucol therapy: a randomized clinical trial. *Circulation* 1996; **94**: I-91.

40. GISSI-Prevenzione Investigators. Dietary supplementation with n-3 polyunsaturated fatty acids and Vitamin E after myocardial infarction: results of the GISSI-Prevenzione trial. *Lancet* 1999; **354**: 447–55.

41. Watanabe K, Sekiya M, Ikeda S, Miyagawa M, Hashida K. Preventive effects of probucol on restenosis after percutaneous transluminal coronary angioplasty. *Am Heart J* 1996; **132**: 23–9.

42. Lee YJ, Daida H, Yokoi H, Miyano H, Takaya J, Sakurai H, Mokuno H, Yamaguchi H. Effectiveness of probucol in preventing restenosis after percutaneous transluminal coronary angioplasty. *Jpn Heart J* 1996; **37**: 327–32.

43. O'Keefe JH, Jr, Stone GW, McCallister BD, Jr, Maddex C, Ligon R, Kacich RL, Kahn J, Cavero PG, Hartzler GO, McCallister BD. Lovastatin plus probucol for prevention of restenosis after percutaneous transluminal coronary angioplasty. *Am J Cardiol* 1996; **77**: 649–52.

44. Stephens NG, Parsons A, Schofield PM, Kelly F, Cheeseman K, Mitchinson MJ. Randomised controlled trial of vitamin E in patients with coronary disease: Cambridge Heart Antioxidant Study (CHAOS). *Lancet* 1996; **347**: 781–6.

3

Physiology and pathophysiology of lipid metabolism

ROBERT H KNOPP

INTRODUCTION

Cholesterol is essential for life. Accordingly, the lipoprotein transport system: (i) delivers cholesterol to the sites where it is required; (ii) recycles cholesterol, so as to not cause any wastage; and (iii) maintains homeostasis. When cholesterol and fat are abundant in the diet and interact with genetic abnormalities to cause hyperlipidemia and atherosclerosis, the idea that cholesterol should be conserved at all is somewhat foreign. Nevertheless, the cholesterol transport system is best understood in these terms.

Cells contain cholesterol and cholesterol ester as part of their surface membrane, and consequently cholesterol is essential for the integrity of all cells and cell renewal. Several organ systems are particularly dependent on the availability of cholesterol, including the central and peripheral nervous systems and steroid-hormone secreting glands including the adrenal, ovaries, testes, and placenta. Red blood cells also contain cholesterol in their surface membranes, and although they are probably no different from other cells in this respect they have a special function in that they circulate and can exchange lipids with other cells and lipoproteins during the course of their lifespan in the intravascular space. Lipoproteins carry out the same function, but with much greater specificity.

NORMAL LIPOPROTEIN METABOLISM

The physiology of lipoprotein transport is illustrated schematically in Figure 3.1.[1] The lipoprotein transport pathway can be divided into exogenous and endogenous compartments. The exogenous pathway comprises the absorption of fatty acids and cholesterol from the intestine and delivery of cholesterol to the liver, while the endogenous pathway comprises the secretion of lipoproteins by the liver, their delivery to peripheral cells, their return to the liver and/or other circulating lipoproteins and excretion in the bile.

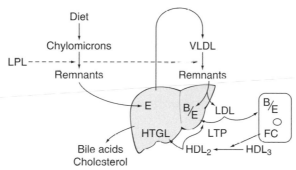

Figure 3.1 *Lipoprotein transport pathway. Exogenous cholesterol is absorbed from the gut and transported to the liver by chylomicron remnants. Endogenous cholesterol is secreted from the liver in the form of VLDL and is degraded to VLDL remnants and LDL. HDL is responsible for reverse cholesterol transport. B/E refers to the LDL receptor, HTGL refers to hepatic (triglyceride) lipase. See text for details. Reproduced with permission from Reference 1.*

The exogenous pathway

CHYLOMICRON FORMATION AND ABSORPTION

After digestion, cholesterol is absorbed with fatty acids and monoglycerides in the form of micelles that are solubilized by components of bile including bile acids, cholesterol and phospholipids found in the biliary effluent. The absorption of cholesterol is regulated, averaging about 50 percent in most individuals but decreasing as the amount of cholesterol ingested increases.[2] Very recently, ABCG5 and ABCG8 proteins have been found to control cholesterol absorption by causing resecretion into the lumen.[3,4] Plant sterols such as sitosterol and sitostanol inhibit cholesterol absorption,[5] except in cases of abnormal ABC proteins where the plant sterols are also absorbed, leading to sitosterolemia, hypercholesterolemia and early atherosclerosis.[4] The new drug ezetimibe also inhibits cholesterol absorption. In addition to cholesterol being absorbed from the diet and from the bile, it can also be manufactured in the gut wall. Cholesterol is largely esterified, and fatty acids are also esterified to form triacylglycerol (triglyceride). These neutral lipids form the core, while phospholipids and apoproteins (apo) B-48, E and C (Figure 3.2) comprise the surface of chylomicrons; this is a common pattern for all lipoproteins. Chylomicrons are absorbed through the lymphatic system and enter the circulation. Only

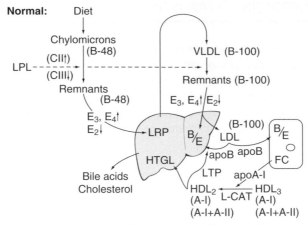

Lp(a) is not involved in metabolism

Figure 3.2 *Apolipoproteins involved in the regulation of lipoprotein transport. Apo B-48 is a structural protein constituent of the chylomicron that does not bind to the LDL receptor. Apo C-II activator and C-III inhibit lipoprotein lipase activity. Apoproteins E3 and E4 bind to the hepatic LDL receptor-related protein (LRP), which takes up the chylomicron remnants. Arrows refer to activation or inhibiton of LPL activty or remnant removal. Apo B-100 is a constituent of VLDL, its remnant and LDL and binds to the LDL receptor. Apoproteins A-I and A-II are constituents of HDL, with A-I facilitating the association with peripheral cells and the initiation of reverse cholesterol transport.*

short- and medium-chain length fatty acids become esterified to form medium-chain triglyceride that can be absorbed directly into the portal circulation.

The clearance of chylomicrons is quite rapid, taking approximately 30 min. However, the absorption of fat is slow and the post-prandial rise and fall of plasma triglyceride concentrations reflects this process, with a peak at approximately 4 h after eating. The significance of this observation is related to observations that post-prandial hypertriglyceridemia is an independent risk factor for coronary artery disease, in addition to its dependency on the fasting triglyceride level, which is itself a cardiovascular disease risk factor (see below).

Once in the circulation, the chylomicrons are degraded by interaction with lipoprotein lipase, a lipolytic enzyme tethered to a variety of cells such as cardiac myocytes, adipose tissue cells, and contractile muscle cells.[6] The lipoprotein lipase enzyme is attached to the capillary endothelium by proteoglycan binding and acts on the chylomicron as it passes through capillaries. This lipolysis within the circulation generates free fatty acids and mono- and diglycerides. Approximately 50 percent of the free fatty acids generated in this manner are absorbed locally, whilst the other 50 percent circulate to the liver, where metabolism proceeds. A cofactor for the lipolytic process is required, apoprotein C-II. By contrast, apoprotein C-III appears to inhibit lipolysis and is a marker for atherosclerosis risk (Figure 3.2).[7,8]

THE CHYLOMICRON REMNANT

Once the triglyceride load of the chylomicron is reduced to a certain point, it takes on the characteristic of the remnant, which is relatively more rich in cholesterol and protein. The relevant protein for the metabolism of the chylomicron remnant is apoprotein E.[9] Apoprotein E is recognized by an low-density lipoprotein (LDL)-like receptor in the liver called the LDL receptor-related protein (LRP). This receptor, while having numerous functions including recognizing and taking up α-macroglobulin, also recognizes the multiple copies of apoprotein E present on the surface of the chylomicron remnant and allows it to be taken up and entered into hepatic metabolism. The specificity of this interaction is very important, since this receptor does not appear to function in any significant degree elsewhere in the body and thus provides for the direct delivery of intestinal cholesterol to the liver where its subsequent metabolism can be highly regulated. Conversely, the apo B-48 of the chylomicron does not recognize the LDL receptor, thus precluding chylomicron remnant uptake by peripheral cells. This scenario differs from glucose and triglyceride fatty acid metabolism, where these energy nutrients can be taken up by any cells in the body, as well as the liver.

Dietary cholesterol has an important effect on hepatic cholesterol metabolism. An increase in cholesterol input via the diet can suppress hepatic cholesterol synthesis and LDL receptor activity. In this way, the liver adjusts to dietary variation in cholesterol input, damping fluctuations in cholesterol supply and thereby maintaining overall body–cholesterol balance. Exceptions exist in the extent to which cholesterol synthesis can be reduced, with 'cholesterol responders' having an excessive rise of plasma cholesterol when ingesting a cholesterol-rich diet. Overall, the amount of cholesterol turned over per day in the body is about 1.2 g, with approximately 10–20 percent of that derived from dietary cholesterol. On average, individuals may ingest 200 to 400 mg of cholesterol daily in an unrestricted diet, and about half of this – or even less – is absorbed (100–200 mg daily). Based on these data, it can be easily seen why restricting cholesterol intake even by 50 percent is unlikely to achieve much benefit because the decrease of 50–100 mg in absorbed dietary cholesterol is small relative to the 1.2 g total daily economy of cholesterol metabolism. On the other hand, inhibiting the combined absorption of dietary and biliary cholesterol can have a more substantial effect on plasma cholesterol, as is seen with ezetimibe.[5,10]

The endogenous pathway of lipoprotein metabolism

VERY LOW–DENSITY LIPOPROTEIN (VLDL) METABOLISM

Lipoproteins appear in the circulation in the form of VLDL from the liver as the point of entry in the endogenous pathway. VLDL is secreted from the liver in various sizes, in association with apoprotein B-100 (see Figure 3.2). The largest and most buoyant VLDL particle is triglyceride-rich and relatively apo B-100 poor, and has limited access to the arterial wall. A more apo B-100 rich, lipid-poor form of VLDL is also secreted; this smaller form is more cholesterol-rich and potentially more atherogenic because it has greater ability to penetrate the endothelial surface. As in the case of metabolism of chylomicrons, VLDL triglyceride is similarly catabolized by lipoprotein lipase (see Figure 3.1).[6] The ability of the body to catabolize VLDL triglyceride can be impaired in the face of chylomicronemia, because most of the lipoprotein lipase will be removing chylomicron triglyceride. Conversely, chylomicronemia can be more likely to develop in the face of endogenous hypertriglyceridemia associated with excessive secretion of VLDL. For this reason, Figure 3.1 shows (diagrammatically) the same enzyme lipoprotein lipase interacting simultaneously with chylomicron and VLDL triglyceride. Apo C-II is again a necessary plasma cofactor for the action of lipoprotein lipase (see Figure 3.2).

THE VLDL REMNANT

As in the case of the exogenous pathway, the progressive removal of VLDL triglyceride leaves a remnant particle that exposes apolipoprotein E on the surface of the particle and allows for its recognition by hepatic receptors. Remnants are recognized by the LDL receptor but also may be recognized by the LRP, which also recognizes the chylomicron remnant. In addition, VLDL receptors have been described which are part of the lipoprotein receptor family and may also have a role to play in the removal of VLDL particles, even before their conversion to the remnant. Nonetheless, much of the remnant lipoprotein passes through the liver in the course of further triglyceride removal and is converted to low-density lipoprotein. This final triglyceride removal step is mediated by hepatic lipase (referred to as HTGL in figures 3.1 and 3.2), which is related to lipoprotein lipase but is specific for hydrolyzing remnant, LDL and HDL triglyceride.[9,11]

LDL METABOLISM

Once LDL is formed, the apo B-100 on its surface is recognized and the entire LDL is removed by LDL receptors on peripheral cells in need of cholesterol for remodeling, for endocrine synthesis by testes, ovary, adrenal and placenta, or is taken up by the liver. Approximately 70 percent of LDL is recycled to the liver, indicating a high degree of reserve in LDL availability for cells in times of high demand such as pregnancy. A plasminogen-like glycopeptide binds to LDL in the plasma to form lipoprotein (a) [Lp(a)], which has no known physiological function. Lp(a) is highly associated with atherosclerosis and thrombosis by enhancing LDL binding to arterial wall and inhibiting the generation of plasmin.[12–14] Small dense LDL, which is also more atherogenic, is generated by an increased activity of hepatic lipase.[11]

HDL METABOLISM

Because cells are constantly remodeling, excess cholesterol, used cholesterol or even oxidized cholesterol may be removed via the reverse cholesterol transport pathway.[15–17] This pathway involves the uptake of free cholesterol by high-density lipoprotein (HDL), involving apoprotein A-I recognition by the ABCA1 transporter protein,[4,17] its esterification by lecithin-cholesterol acyltransferase and movement to the lipoprotein core (the lipoprotein 'baggage compartment') (Figure 3.3) and its recycling either to the liver (mediated by hepatic lipase) or to LDL and VLDL via cholesterol ester transfer protein (CETP). Many steps are involved in this process, and new receptors and points of regulation are continually being discovered.[4,17] Apoproteins A-I and A-II are components of HDL (see Figure 3.2); most important of these is apoprotein A-I, and its synthesis by the liver and incorporation into HDL are essential to the function of HDL in of reverse cholesterol transport. HDL also

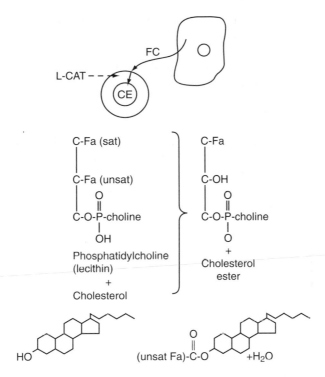

Figure 3.3 *Lecithin-cholesterol acyltransferase (L-CAT) physiology. L-CAT transfers a fatty acid from lecithin to cholesterol to form a cholesterol ester. This esterification converts cholesterol from a polar surface lipid to a neutral lipid which migrates to the core 'baggage compartment' of HDL and enables small HDL (HDL$_3$) to enlarge to HDL$_2$. This maturation of HDL allows reverse cholesterol transport to proceed.*

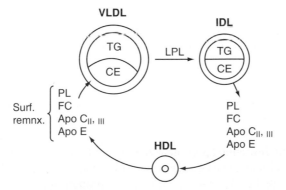

Figure 3.4 *Exchange of surface remnants (surf. remnx.) between VLDL or IDL and HDL. Surface remnants consist of phospholipids (PL), free cholesterol (FC), apoproteins C-II and C-II and apo E. All of these constituents are polar and attached to the surface of the lipoprotein particles. As VLDL is degraded to a remnant by lipoprotein lipase (LPL), it becomes smaller and the surface coat shrinks, transferring these constituents to HDL. In hypertriglyceridemia, less transfer occurs to HDL, contributing to low HDL levels.*

serves as a reservoir for surface remnants of VLDL metabolism (Figure 3.4). Surface remnants (free cholesterol, phospholipid and apoproteins C and E) are shed as the VLDL particle becomes smaller under the action of lipoprotein lipase and freely exchange to and from HDL. HDL also carries natural anti-oxidants that can help defend LDL against oxidative stress. A deficiency of the ABCA1 transporter protein causes a failure of HDL generation, with extremely low HDL-cholesterol (HDL-C) levels of 1–4 mg/dL, a condition known as Tangier disease.[17]

THE FIVE PRIMARY LIPID DISORDERS (FIGURE 3.5; TABLE 3.1)[18]

Hypertriglyceridemia/familial hypertriglyceridemia (HTG/FHTG)

CHILDHOOD FORM

The most extreme (and clear-cut) example of familial hypertriglyceridemia is that seen in childhood due to homozygous deficiency of lipoprotein lipase activity.[6,19] These individuals have mutations in the LPL gene or its promoter segment, and this results in 10 percent or less of normal lipoprotein lipase activity. Under these circumstances, individuals will have extreme intolerance to ingested fat, and for this reason this condition was known in the past as fat-induced hypertriglyceridemia. These chylomicrons have poor access to the arterial wall because of their large size. They can cause pancreatitis if triglyceride levels exceed 2000 mg/dL (see below).

ADULT FORM

In adulthood, familial hypertriglyceridemia is usually caused by an overproduction of VLDL by the liver, but it may also be caused by a partial deficiency of lipoprotein lipase (see Figure 3.1) or rarely the activator protein apo C-II.[6] This form of VLDL overproduction is due to excessive formation of plasma triglyceride with a normal amount of apoprotein B accompanying the formed VLDL particle. LPL deficiency can lead to the same type of VLDL accumulation. In these circumstances, the VLDL particle is very triglyceride-rich, very large and very buoyant, and also passes poorly through the endothelial barrier into the arterial wall. These 'large and fluffy' VLDL are considered to be non-atherogenic or benign, and are associated with the type of hypertriglyceridemia that is seen, for example, with excessive alcohol ingestion or estrogen therapy.[20] Clinically, the only way to insure that the condition is not atherogenic is to examine the patient and the family history for evidence of vascular disease.

An animal model of this non-atherogenic hyperlipidemia is seen in the cholesterol-fed rabbit, ordinarily a classical model of atherosclerosis. However, if the rabbit is made diabetic simultaneously, then lipoprotein lipase activity is reduced, the VLDL particles become very large, and atherosclerosis no longer occurs. Unfortunately, this scenario does not apply to most secondary causes of hyper-triglyceridemia in humans, including thiazide or beta-blocker therapy or diabetes or nephrotic syndrome. These atherogenic conditions are discussed elsewhere.

In summary, FHTG/HTG has two etiologies: (i) a deficiency of lipoprotein lipase activity; or (ii) an excess production of buoyant VLDL particles. If familial, the

Table 3.1 *Primary lipoprotein disorders amenable to treatment with diet and drug therapy[a]*

Disorder	Mechanisms	Complications	Treatment[b]
Familial hypertriglyceridemia[c]	Decreased serum triglyceride removal resulting from decreased LPL activity Increased hepatic secretion of triglyceride-rich VLDL	Pancreatitis at triglyceride concentrations >2000 mg per deciliter (22.6 mmol/liter); low risk of CAD	Diet and weight loss Fibrate Nicotinic acid n–3 fatty acids Oxandrolone
Familial combined hyperlipidemia[c]	Increased hepatic secretion of apolipoprotein B – containing VLDL and conversion to LDL Accumulation of VLDL, LDL, or both, depending on efficiency of their removal	CAD, PVD, stroke	Diet and weight loss Statin Nicotinic acid Fibrate[d] Exetimibe
Remnant removal disease (familial dysbetalipo-proteinemia)	Increased secretion of VLDL Impaired removal of remnant lipoproteins resulting from homozygosity ($\varepsilon_2/\varepsilon_3$) or heterozygosity ($\varepsilon_2/\varepsilon_3$ or $\varepsilon_2/\varepsilon_4$) for apolipoprotein E ε_2	PVD, CAD, stroke	Diet, weight loss Fibrate[d] Nicotinic acid Statin
Familial or polygenic hypercholesterolemia	Diminished LDL-receptor activity Defective apolipoprotein B that is poorly recognized by LDL receptor	CAD, occasionally PVD, stroke	Diet Statin Bile-acid-binding resin Nicotinic acid Ezetimibe Fibrate
Familial hypoalphalipo-proteinemia (low HDL syndrome)[e]	Diminished apolipoprotein A–I formation, increased removal, increased CETP or hepatic lipase activity	CAD, PVD (may be associated with hypertriglyceridemia)	Exercise and weight loss Nicotinic acid Fibrate[d] Statin

[a]LPL denotes lipoprotein lipase, VLDL very-low-density lipoprotein, CAD coronary artery disease, PVD peripheral vascular disease, HDL high-density lipoprotein, and CETP cholesterol-ester transfer protein.
[b]The treatments may be given alone or in combination; the primary treatment is listed first, followed by other treatments in decreasing order of importance.
[c]Diabetes mellitus can greatly exacerbate the condition. The hyperlipidemia of diabetes is closest mechanistically to familial combined hyperlipidemia.
[d]Combined treatment with a fibrate and a statin can increase the risk of myopathy.
[e]This disorder is characterized by low concentrations of HDL cholesterol.
From the *New England Journal of Medicine* (Reference 10) with permission.

condition is characterized by a consistent excess of triglyceride without major cholesterol or LDL-cholesterol (LDL-C) elevations in the proband as well as relatives. HTG/FHTG is not usually associated with atherosclerosis (absence of family history of coronary artery disease is another important clue). However, HTG/FHTG can become clinically very important if the plasma triglyceride exceeds 2000 mg/dL,

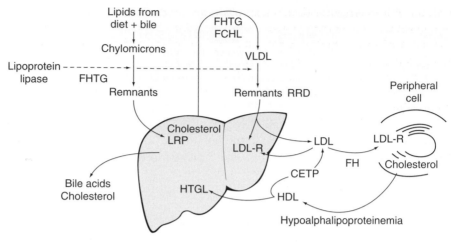

Figure 3.5 *Pathways of lipid transport. Cholesterol is absorbed from the intestine and transported to the liver by chylomicron remnants, which are taken up by the low-density lipoprotein (LDL)-receptor-related protein (LRP). Hepatic cholesterol enters the circulation as very-low-density lipoprotein (VLDL) and is metabolized to remnant lipoproteins after lipoprotein lipase removes triglyceride. The remnant lipoproteins are removed by LDL receptors (LDL-R), or are further metabolized to LDL and then removed by these receptors. Cholesterol is transported from peripheral cells to the liver by high-density lipoprotein (HDL). Cholesterol is recycled to LDL and VLDL by cholesterol-ester transport protein (CETP), or is taken up in the liver by hepatic lipase. Cholesterol is excreted in the bile. The points in the process that cause the five primary lipoprotein disorders – familial hypertriglyceridemia (FHTG), familial combined hyperlipidemia (FCHL), remnant removal disease (RRD; also known as familial dysbetalipoproteinemia), familial hypercholesterolemia (FH) and hypoalpha-lipoproteinemia – are shown. The effects of drug therapy can also be understood from these pathways. Statins decrease the synthesis of cholesterol and the secretion of VLDL, and increase the activity of LDL-R. Bile acid-binding resins increase the secretion of bile acids. Nicotinic acid decreases the secretion of VLDL and the formation of LDL, and increases the formation of HDL. Fibrates decrease the secretion of VLDL and increase the activity of lipoprotein lipase, thereby increasing the removal of triglycerides. Ezetimibe decreases cholesterol absorption from the gut. (Adapted from Knopp.[18])*

which is the threshold for the causation of pancreatitis. A plasma triglyceride level of 1000 mg/dL (11.3 mM) or higher is a warning sign, since a triglyceride level of 2000 mg/dL (22.6 mM) can be reached quickly with very little further increase in hepatic VLDL production due to near-saturation of the LPL removal mechanism.

Combined hyperlipidemia/familial combined hyperlipidemia (CHL/FCHL)

This category of hyperlipidemia is the most important in terms of numbers of persons affected. These conditions have the common characteristic of over-production of lipoproteins by the liver, primarily in the form of VLDL of moderate size and with less triglyceride and relatively more apoprotein B and cholesterol than seen in FHTG.[21] Overproduction of VLDL can occur as a primary disorder known as familial combined hyperlipidemia, which derives from diminished degradation of apo B within the liver and an oversecretion of apo B-rich VLDL. These particles are believed to have access to the arterial wall and can be atherogenic in their own right. It is also possible that such VLDL can even have a direct toxic effect on the endothelium.

However, not all familial combined hyperlipidemic individuals manifest with an excess in plasma triglyceride levels, and this accounts for the great confusion associated with this category.[22] As shown in Figure 3.5, an excess of VLDL secretion can also lead to an excess of remnant lipoprotein or an excess of LDL. Thus, the manifestations of FCHL or its related secondary overproduction disorders (diabetes, obesity, insulin resistance, steroid hormone therapy, isotretinoin administration) depends on the relative efficiency of removal of each of the three apo B-containing particles; that is, VLDL, remnants or LDL (see Table 3.1). Therefore, an overproduction of lipoprotein entering the bloodstream in the form of VLDL can manifest as a VLDL increase, a remnant increase, an LDL increase, or combinations thereof. In lipid terms, this scenario means that individuals with either CHL or FCHL can present as having high triglyceride, high cholesterol, or high cholesterol and triglyceride. In the case of combined elevations of cholesterol and triglyceride levels, the elevations may be due to an excess of VLDL and LDL together, or to an excess of remnant lipoprotein, which bears equal amounts of cholesterol and triglyceride in a single particle.

In summary, there are several reasons for the name 'combined or familial combined hyperlipidemia.' First, the name connotes hyperlipidemia that can present with different combinations or manifestations of hyperlipidemia, high cholesterol, high triglyceride, or both. Second, expression of the hyperlipidemia can change in a given individual. For instance, fibric acid treatment, fish oil therapy or weight loss decrease the triglyceride and raise the LDL-C, whereas diabetes or a high-carbohydrate diet do the reverse. Third, varied forms of hyperlipidemia can present among family members, one with high triglyceride, one with high cholesterol, and/or another with both elevated. A final clinical clue is the presence of premature cardiovascular disease in the patient or among first- and second-degree relatives. Among these manifestations in the patient proband are premature arcus senilis, carotid or ileo-femoral bruits, a harsh aortic ejection murmur due to aortic calcification, or missing or asymmetric foot pulses. The essential therapeutic point is that combined elevations of cholesterol and triglyceride require combined lipid-lowering therapy, ideally a reductase inhibitor and niacin, or failing that a reductase inhibitor and fibrate, observing appropriate myositis precaution.[18]

In any of these conditions which are associated with lipoprotein overproduction from the liver, coexistence with obesity, syndrome X, insulin resistance or frank diabetes can exaggerate hyperlipidemia greatly. Especially in the case of diabetes, offending drugs and nephrotic syndrome, lipoprotein overproduction and/or a simultaneous reduction in lipoprotein lipase activity due to the impaired effectiveness of insulin can lead to massive hypertriglyceridemia and pancreatitis as discussed above under HTG/FHTG. Thus, individuals at risk for pancreatitis are not only those with hypertriglyceridemia (HTG/FHTG) but also those with CHL/FCHL complicated by an additional disorder that aggravates lipoprotein overproduction or impair triglyceride-rich lipoprotein removal.

Remnant removal disease (RRD)

Although this condition has already been introduced as one of the manifestations of CHL/FCHL, RRD has special diagnostic requirements and a different approach to therapy such that it is usually considered in its own diagnostic category.[9,12] RRD is also known by other names such as familial dysbetalipoproteinemia or Type III hyperlipidemia, but RRD is the most descriptive.

The diagnostic problem arises when one is confronted with combined elevations of cholesterol and triglyceride which can signify a combined elevation of VLDL and LDL or a primary elevation of remnant lipoprotein. Diagnostic testing involves identifying cholesterol enrichment of the remnant lipoprotein itself or the abnormal apoprotein (apo E2) that is poorly recognized by the LDL or LRP receptors in the liver and causes remnant accumulation in the blood (Box 3.1; see Figure 3.2).

Direct lipoprotein measurement is required to detect the remnant particle. This procedure allows calculation of the VLDL-cholesterol to total plasma triglyceride ratio which, if greater than 0.3, indicates an excess of remnant lipoprotein in the VLDL range. An average ratio is 0.20. If this VLDL is run on gel electrophoresis, it has the electrophoretic characteristics of both VLDL (pre-β band) and LDL (β band) and is therefore known as β-migrating VLDL. A more modern form of detection involves identification of apoprotein isoforms in the homozygous (E2/E2) or heterozygous (E2/E3 or E2/E4) forms. The homozygous and heterozygous forms are associated with more or less severe manifestations of remnant accumulation, respectively. Rarer apoprotein E mutations may not follow the E2 genotype and may manifest as a dominant form, but the apo E2 recessive form is the most common in

---

Box 3.1 *Diagnostic characteristics of remnant removal disease (RRD)*

Ultracentrifugation: (direct separation of VLDL and LDL at density 1.006)
- VLDL-C/total triglyceride ratio exceeds 0.30
- An average (normal) VLDL-C/total triglyceride ratio is 0.20 and is the basis for estimating VLDL-C from the concentration of total triglyceride (triglyceride ÷ 5)

Electrophoresis:
- *Whole plasma*: a broad beta band is observed encompassing pre-beta and beta bands
- *VLDL isolated by centrifugation*: remnant migration is seen in both the VLDL (pre-beta) as well as LDL (beta) regions; therefore the remnant is designated as beta-migrating VLDL

Apoprotein E identification: by isoelectric focusing (old) or genotyping or immunoblotting (new)
- Apo E2/E2: homozygous for RRD
- Apo E2/E3 or E2/E4: heterozygous for RRD
- Apo E3/E3: wild-type
- Apo E3/E4 or E4/E4: associated with increased LDL and CVD

the general population. Another important feature is a low LDL level. When remnants accumulate, little LDL is formed; in fact, in the absence of excess lipoprotein production associated with CHL/FHCL, individuals with the apo E2 isoform have no hyperlipidemia and the low LDL levels extend longevity.

In summary, RRD is an unusual manifestation of hepatic lipid overproduction combined with a deficiency of remnant clearance. This condition is highly atherogenic, especially to the peripheral vasculature. Fortunately, it is not common and is usually very sensitive to therapy.

Polygenic or familial hypercholesterolemia (PFH/FH)

The classic form of familial hypercholesterolemia is due to a deficiency of LDL receptor activity, which impairs the removal of LDL, both by peripheral cells and the liver.[12] Known mutations in the LDL receptor gene now number over 300. Individuals with heterozygous FH number 1 in 500 in the population and have approximately double the LDL-C level due to a 50 percent reduction in LDL receptor activity; thus their LDL-C levels are typically 240–260 mg/dL, compared to an average LDL level of 130 mg/dL. Homozygotes with genetic deficits in both LDL receptor genes are rare, except in cases of familial consanguinity or highly inbred populations such as seen in Lebanon, Quebec, and Japan. It also appears that a deficiency of LDL receptor activity is associated with an enhanced endogenous production of cholesterol and export into the circulation.

Polygenic familial hypercholesterolemia (PFH) runs in families, is not specifically associated with a classical single gene mutation, but has multiple genetic inputs. Such individuals are difficult to distinguish from those with FH, except by the use of genetic studies. The differentiation has little practical therapeutic significance except that such individuals are typically less severely affected.

A companion condition that is indistinguishable from familial heterozygous or homozygous hypercholesterolemia is due to a defective apo B. An abnormal structure of apo B in the receptor binding region results in a failure to recognize the LDL receptor. Otherwise, all manifestations tend to be the same as in FH, including severe hypercholesterolemia, early onset of atherosclerosis, tendinous xanthomas, and arcus senilis. These individuals respond to therapy as well as those with inherited LDL receptor deficits. To date, there is no practical clinical reason to distinguish this condition from the other forms of FH.

Low LDL syndromes (hypobetalipoproteinemia)

The converse of high LDL levels or FH is familial hypobetalipoproteinemia, which is associated with truncations of various lengths in the apo B molecule and an inability to form normal amounts of VLDL. Defects result in an impaired secretion of VLDL and impaired formation of remnants and LDL. Total LDL and cholesterol levels are strikingly low. Surprisingly, individuals are not adversely affected by these deficiencies and have greater longevity as a result.

Individuals who have a total deficiency of apo B formation cannot form chylomicrons and cannot absorb fat and do not transport cholesterol in VLDL or

LDL. These individuals have the classical abetalipoproteinemia associated with fat malabsorption, vitamin E deficiency, retinitis pigmentosa, crenated red cells and central nervous system manifestations such as ataxia. The central nervous system symptoms are due to the vitamin E deficiency. Short of fat malabsorption and vitamin A, D, E and K deficiency, it appears that individuals who are deficient in apo B-containing lipoprotein transport (VLDL, remnant, LDL) do not suffer any meaningful deficiency in cholesterol availability for cell remodeling or steroid hormone formation, since HDL can also supply cholesterol to cells as well as remove it. It is now believed that HDL-C delivery to cells is accomplished by the scavenger receptor SR-B1. As an example, such individuals experience no difficulty in maintaining a normal full-term pregnancy, though plasma steroid hormone levels may be slightly reduced.

Low HDL syndromes (hypoalphalipoproteinemia)

The term hypoalphalipoproteinemia derives from the alpha migration of HDL in gel electrophoresis systems. Numerous metabolic defects can result in minor or major reductions in HDL.[15,16] One category of abnormalities results from a reduction in the formation of the building blocks of HDL. These include a diminished hepatic secretion of apoprotein A-I due to various gene defects in the apo A-I gene. A secondary cause involves a diminished transfer of VLDL surface remnants (free cholesterol, phospholipid, apoproteins C and E) to HDL (see Figure 3.4). Such individuals usually have normal apo A-I levels.

Another category of low HDL is related to defects in the reverse cholesterol transport regulatory process. These disorders include an inability to move cholesterol from the interior of the cell to the surface, or an inability of the cholesterol to be taken up by HDL (as is seen in Tangier disease).[17] Both conditions lead to a failure of formation of HDL and extremely low HDL-C levels in the range of 1–4 mg/dL. Free cholesterol accepted onto the HDL particle from the surface of peripheral cells is esterified by the enzyme lecithin cholesterol acyl transferase (LCAT) (see Figure 3.3). The discovery of this enzyme led to the idea of a reverse cholesterol transport pathway. In the case of a lack of LCAT activity, an excess of free cholesterol accumulates in membranes and all lipoproteins, beginning with HDL. In the absence of cholesterol esterification, free cholesterol accumulates on the surface of the cells. The absence of esterified cholesterol prevents the maturation of nascent HDL from disks to a spherical form where the neutral cholesterol ester accumulates in the core. Once mature, HDL in the form of HDL_2 releases cholesterol to the liver through hepatic lipase activity. People with high hepatic lipase activity have low HDL-C levels. In addition, HDL-C ester is transferred to LDL and VLDL in exchange for triglyceride via cholesterol ester transfer protein, or CETP (Figure 3.6). Individuals with high CETP activity would tend to have high LDL and low HDL levels. Similarly, hypertriglyceridemia can favor CETP-mediated lipid exchange leading to low HDL-C levels (Figure 3.6). Once the cholesterol is removed from the HDL particle, the triglyceride contained in HDL can be degraded (also by hepatic lipase), and the remodeled HDL can return to the peripheral cells for uptake of cholesterol again. Thus, the protein structure of HDL is preserved for reuse.

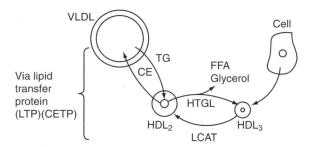

Figure 3.6 *Cholesterol ester (CE)/triglyceride (TG) exchange by lipid transfer protein (LTP), also known as cholesterol ester transfer protein (CETP). Once triglyceride has been transferred from VLDL to HDL, hepatic lipase (hepatic triglyceride lipase or HTGL) breaks down HDL-TG into free fatty acids (FFA) and glycerol. By this mechanism, HDL is reduced in size from HDL$_2$ to HDL$_3$ and can pick up more free cholesterol from cells to initiate a new round of reverse cholesterol transport.*

In summary, the physiology of reverse cholesterol transport involves multiple steps with multiple mechanisms for abnormalities. These conditions are broadly classified into six categories in Box 3.2.

UNUSUAL INTERACTIONS AMONG THE GENETIC FORMS OF HYPERLIPIDEMIA

Though the five treatable forms of hyperlipidemia are considered as single discrete entities, combinations of these disorders are to be expected, and do in fact exist. Thus, an individual who has RRD could also have FH. The presentation in this instance is an extreme cholesterol elevation with hypertriglyceridemia. Marked improvement is seen in the triglyceride elevation with fibric acid therapy, but a marked elevation in LDL results. Thus, treatment of the hypertriglyceridemia reveals the underlying hypercholestcrolemia, which can be very severe. Such individuals will have multiple cholesterol deposits in plantar and skin surfaces on the extensor tendons and large tendons. As mentioned elsewhere, severe hypertriglyceridemias can occur, particularly when diabetes is associated with FHTG, FCHL or RRD. These individuals are all predisposed to eruptive xanthoma formation, and pancreatitis.

Another common interaction is that the familial hypertriglyceridemias are associated with low HDL levels, which are due to the lack of surface remnant transfer from VLDL to HDL. These individuals will tend to have normal HDL apoprotein levels; that is, a normal apoprotein A-I level, typically around 130 mg/dL.

SUMMARY

The transport of lipoproteins in the body is divided into exogenous and endogenous pathways, with the liver as the 'grand central terminal' for lipoprotein lipid uptake, formation, and degradation. Aspects of these pathways are reviewed in Figures 3.1,

---

Box 3.2   *Causes of low plasma HDL levels*

Low apo A-I synthesis:
- A variety of defects in the apo A-I gene

Hypertriglyceridemia:
- Reduced transfer of VLDL surface remnants to HDL due to retarded VLDL catabolism

Abnormal cell delivery of cholesterol:
- Poor movement of cholesterol to the cell surface
- Poor recognition of apo A-I or phospholipid cholesterol acceptors in the plasma with poor generation of HDL (Tangier disease)

LCAT deficiency:
- Failure of cholesterol to be esterified so that it does not accumulate in the core of the HDL particle, impeding reverse transport of cholesterol in any quantity

Hepatic lipase overactivity:
- Increased HDL-cholesterol uptake in the liver generates cholesterol ester-poor HDL

CETP activity is increased:
- A cholesterol-poor HDL is generated and VLDL-C and LDL-cholesterol levels are elevated as increased amounts of cholesterol ester are transferred from HDL in exchange for triglyceride

---

3.2, and 3.5. The five main categories of lipid disorders are also listed in Table 3.1. Many of these disorders are single base defects but occur at multiple sites within the given gene. Less extreme polygenic forms of all of these disorders exist or are likely to exist. Furthermore, genetic forms of polygenic or monogenic nature can cosegregate, yielding combined or hybrid forms of hyperlipidemia. The implication of this heterogeneity of the lipoprotein disorders is that gene therapy may require more precise analysis of the lipoprotein regulatory genome than has heretofore been considered to be necessary or desirable. On the other hand, the rewards of such diagnostic precision may be great if gene therapy can be completely curative. The present alternative – which itself is considered to be quite advanced – is the long-term multi-drug therapy of severe lipoprotein disorders.

REFERENCES

1. Knopp RH. The effects of oral contraceptives and postmenopausal estrogens on lipoprotein physiology and atherosclerosis. In: Halbe HW, Rekers H, eds. *Oral Contraception into the 1990's*. Carnforth, UK: Parthenon Publishing; 1989: 31–45.
2. Ostlund RE, Jr, Bosner MS, Stenson WF. Cholesterol absorption efficiency declines at moderate dietary doses in normal human subjects. *J Lipid Res* 1999; **40**: 1453–8.
3. Berge KE, Tian H, Graf GA, Yu L, Grishin NV, Schultz J, *et al*. Accumulation of dietary cholesterol in sitosterolemia caused by mutations in adjacent ABC transporters. *Science* 2000; **290**: 1771–5.

4. Allayee H, Laffitte BA, Lusis AJ. Biochemistry. An absorbing study of cholesterol. *Science* 2000; **290**: 1709–11.

5. Miettinen TA, Puska P, Gylling H, Vanhanen H, Vartiainen E. Reduction of serum cholesterol with sitostanol-ester margarine in a mildly hypercholesterolemic population. *N Engl J Med* 1995; **333**: 1308–12.

6. Brunzell JD. Familial lipoprotein lipase deficiency and other causes of the chylomicronemia syndrome. In: Scriver CR, Beaudet AL, Sly WS, Valle D, eds. *The Metabolic Basis of Inherited Disease.* 7th edn. New York: McGraw-Hill; 1995: 1913–32.

7. Waterworth DM, Ribalta J, Nicaud V, Dallongeville J, Humphries SE, Talmud P. ApoCIII gene variants modulate postprandial response to both glucose and fat tolerance tests. *Circulation* 1999; **99**: 1872–7.

8. Brown B, Zhao X-Q, Chait A, Fisher L, Cheung M, Morse J, *et al*. Simvastatin and niacin, antioxidant vitamins, or the combination for the prevention of coronary disease. *N Engl J Med* 2001; **345**: 1583–92.

9. Mahley RW. Apolipoprotcin E: cholesterol transport protein with expanding role in cell biology. *Science* 1988; **240**: 622–30.

10. Bays HE, Moore PB, Drehobl MA, Rosenblatt S, Toth PD, Dujovne CA, *et al*. Effectiveness and tolerability of ezetimibe in patients with primary hypercholesterolemia: pooled analysis of two phase II studies. *Clin Ther* 2001; **23**: 1209–30.

11. Zambon A, Hokanson JE, Brown BG, Brunzell JD. Evidence for a new pathophysiological mechanism for coronary artery disease regression: hepatic lipase-mediated changes in LDL density. *Circulation* 1999; **99**: 1959–64.

12. Havel RJ, Rapaport E. Management of primary hyperlipidemia [published erratum appears in *N Engl J Med* 1995 Aug 17; 333(7): 467]. *N Engl J Med* 1995; **332**: 1491–8.

13. Summary of the second report of the National Cholesterol Education Program (NCEP) Expert Panel on Detection, Evaluation, and Treatment of High Blood Cholesterol in Adults (Adult Treatment Panel II). *JAMA* 1993; **269**: 3015–23.

14. Executive Summary of The Third Report of The National Cholesterol Education Program (NCEP) Expert Panel on Detection, Evaluation, And Treatment of High Blood Cholesterol In Adults (Adult Treatment Panel III). *JAMA* 2001; **285**: 2486–97.

15. Fielding CJ, Fielding PE. Molecular physiology of reverse cholesterol transport. *J Lipid Res* 1995; **36**: 211–28.

16. Oram JF, Yokoyama S. Apolipoprotein-mediated removal of cellular cholesterol and phospholipids. *J Lipid Res* 1996; **37**: 2473–91.

17. Brooks-Wilson A, Marcil M, Clee SM, Zhang LH, Roomp K, van Dam M, *et al*. Mutations in ABC1 in Tangier disease and familial high-density lipoprotein deficiency. *Nature Genet* 1999; **22**: 336–45.

18. Knopp RH. Drug treatment of lipid disorders. *N Engl J Med* 1999; 341: 498–511.

19. Brunzell JD, Bierman EL. Chylomicronemia syndrome. Interaction of genetic and acquired hypertriglyceridemia. *Med Clin North Am* 1982; **66**: 455–68.

20. Ginsberg HN. Is hypertriglyceridemia a risk factor for atherosclerotic cardiovascular disease? A simple question with a complicated answer. *Ann Intern Med* 1997; **126**: 912–14.

21. Chait A, Albers JJ, Brunzell JD. Very low density lipoprotein overproduction in genetic forms of hypertriglyceridemia. *Eur J Clin Invest* 1980; **10**: 17–22.

22. Goldstein JL, Schrott HG, Hazzard WR, Bierman EL, Motulsky A. Hyperlipidemia in coronary heart disease. II. Genetic analysis of lipid levels in 176 families and delineation of a new inherited disorder, combined hyperlipidemia. *J Clin Invest* 1973; **52**: 1544–68.

4

Secondary causes of hyperlipidemia

SYLVIA VELA

INTRODUCTION

The clinical evaluation of any patient with hyperlipidemia should first involve the exclusion of secondary or acquired causes. Secondary causes of hyperlipidemia often produce an atherogenic lipid profile that places patients at risk of coronary heart disease. Alternatively, acquired causes may result in severe hypertriglyceridemia that can predispose patients to acute pancreatitis. Most importantly, treatment of the underlying cause can often reverse or improve the abnormal lipid profile, obviating or minimizing the need for lipid-lowering medications. Thus, a thorough search for an underlying cause of hyperlipidemia can uncover previously unsuspected disease and can be productive as well as cost-effective when managing these patients.

A comprehensive list of acquired secondary causes of hyperlipidemia is provided in Table 4.1. while specific phenotypes and dyslipidemia are detailed in Table 4.2. The most common factors resulting in induced lipid abnormalities are diabetes mellitus and medications/drugs. This review will address the mechanisms (if known) and significance of some of the more common offenders.

DIABETES MELLITUS

The most common cause of secondary hyperlipidemia is diabetes mellitus. Diabetes induces a state of dyslipidemia, with potential derangements in lipoprotein

Table 4.1 *Acquired secondary causes of hyperlipidemia*

Factor	Cause	Change
Diet	Starvation	↑C
	Weight gain	↑TG
	Weight loss	↓TG, ↑HDL
Drugs	Alcohol	↑TG, ↑HDL
	Alpha blockers	↑HDL
	Amiodarone	↑C
	Anabolic steroids	↑C, ↓HDL
	Anti-epileptics: (phenobarbitone, phenytoin, carbamazepine)	↑HDL
	Anti-psychotics (olanzapine, clozapine)	↑TG
	Beta-blockers:	
	Selective	↑TG, ↓HDL
	Non-selective	↑TG, ↓HDL
	With ISA	↔TG, ↔HDL
	With α activity	↔TG, ↔HDL
	Cyclosporine	↑C, ↑LDL
	Didanosine	↑TG
	Diuretics:	
	Loop	↑C, ↑LDL, ↔TG, ↔HDL
	Thiazides	↑C, ↑LDL, ↑TG, ↔HDL
	Potassium-sparing	↔C, ↔LDL, ↔TG, ↓HDL
	Estrogen	↑C, ↑TG, ↑HDL, ↓LDL
	Fish oil	↓TG, ↑LDL
	Glucocorticoids	↑C, ↑TG, ↑HDL, ↑LDL
	Progestins	↑C, ↓HDL
	Protease inhibitors	↑TG, ↑Lp(a)
	Retinoids	↑C and TG, ↓HDL
	Tamoxifen	↑TG and HDL, ↓LDL
Diseases/ conditions	Acromegaly	↑TG
	Anorexia nervosa	↑C
	Burns	↑TG
	Chlorinated hydrocarbon insecticides	↑C, ↑HDL
	Cholestasis	↑C (Lp-X)
	Chronic renal failure	↑TG, ↓HDL
	Cigarette smoking	↑TG, ↓HDL
	Diabetes mellitus type I	↑TG
	Diabetes mellitus type II	↑TG, ↓HDL
	Glycogen storage diseases	↑TG
	Growth hormone deficiency	↑C
	Hepatitis	↑C, ↑TG
	Hyperandrogenism in women	↑TG, ↓HDL
	Hypothyroidism	↑C and /or TG
	Lipodystrophy	↑TG
	Myelomatosis (IgA, IgG)	↑C
	Nephrotic syndrome	↑C, ↑TG, ↓HDL
	Obesity	↑TG, ↓HDL
	Polyclonal gammopathy	↑TG
	Porphyria (acute intermittent)	↑C
	Pregnancy	↑C, ↑TG
	Systemic lupus erythematosus	↑TG
	Syndrome X	↑TG, ↓HDL
	Transplantation	↑C, ↑TG

Table 4.2 *Specific phenotypes and dyslipidemia*

Lipoprotein	Phenotype	Dyslipidemia	Secondary cause
Chylomicrons	I	LPL deficiency	Dysglobulinemia
		Apo C2 deficiency	Diabetes mellitus
LDL	IIa	Familial hypercholesterolemia Familial defective B-100 Polygenic hypercholesterolemia Familial combined hyperlipidemia Lp(a) excess	Renal disease Nephrotic syndrome Hypothyroidism Cushing's syndrome Dysglobulinemia Acute intermittent porphyria Cholestatic liver disease
LDL and VLDL	IIb	Familial combined hyperlipidemia Hyperapobetalipoproteinemia	Nephrotic syndrome Hypothyroidism Dysglobulinemia Cushing's syndrome Glucocorticoid use Stress-induced
Remnants	III	Familial dysbetalipoproteinemia	Diabetes mellitus Hypothyroidism Dysglobulinemia
VLDL	IV	Familial hypertriglyceridemia Hypertriglyceridemia with low HDL Familial combined hyperlipidemia	Diabetes mellitus Dysglobulinemias Uremia Hypothyroidism Nephrotic syndrome Chronic renal disease Estrogen Glucocorticoids Long-term ethanol use Stress-induced
Chylomicrons and VLDL	V	Familial hypertriglyceridemia Multiple defect hyperlipidemia Partial LPL deficiency Partial apo C-2 deficiency Apo C-3 inhibitor	Diabetes mellitus Dysglobulinemia Estrogen Pregnancy Nephrotic syndrome
Lp(a)	NA	Lp(a) excess	Chronic renal disease Diabetes mellitus Protease inhibitors
HDL	NA	Primary hypoalphalipoproteinemia	Cigarette smoking Obesity Physical inactivity Androgens Beta-blockers

metabolism affecting virtually all of the lipoprotein classes. Most treated diabetics have relatively normal lipid profiles; however, mild to moderate elevations in triglycerides or total cholesterol are more frequent in the diabetic population compared to the normal population; low high-density lipoprotein (HDL) is common. The frequency and severity of the lipid abnormality varies with the type of diabetes; that is, Type 1 versus Type 2 diabetes.

Elevated triglycerides are frequently observed in newly diagnosed or inadequately treated diabetics or untreated patients with ketosis and hyperglycemia, due to higher synthetic rates of very low-density lipoprotein (VLDL) by the liver, as well as delayed clearance by adipose tissue and muscle.[1] Diabetic dyslipidemia is most often seen in patients with Type 2 diabetes and insulin resistance.[2] Levels of low-density lipoprotein (LDL) are usually normal, but triglycerides are elevated and HDL is low. Small, dense LDL particles are an additional part of the syndrome, and this results in a more atherogenic profile despite the relatively normal LDL levels. Triglycerides can be severely elevated (as high as 10 000 mg/dL), especially in patients with an underlying genetic metabolic defect compounded by a reduction in lipoprotein lipase (LPL) activity in insulin deficiency. In the setting of severe hyperglycemia, lipoprotein lipase activity may be reduced, and this contributes to the excess of chylomicrons, VLDL, and remnants.[3] Both glucose and free fatty acids provide the substrate for synthesis of VLDL-cholesterol secretion. Aggressive treatment of the hyperglycemia and/or use of insulin restores the activity of the LPL enzyme and can improve and even normalize the lipid profile. Diabetics who also have a genetic hyperlipoproteinemia may not achieve normalization of the profile.

Concentrations of LDL are typically not elevated in Type 2 diabetics, but may very well have abnormal composition.[3,4] Triglyceride-rich LDL, enrichment with unesterified cholesterol, small dense LDL and glycosylated LDL have all been described in diabetics with hypertriglyceridemia.[5,6] Delayed clearance of LDL particles allowing excessive oxidation has also been demonstrated, and this potentially increases the atherogenic potential of the lipoprotein. In addition, despite normal levels of LDL-cholesterol (LDL-C), almost half of all diabetics have elevated apoprotein B which has been associated with cardiovascular disease.[2,7]

High-density lipoprotein or HDL-cholesterol (HDL-C) is frequently reduced due to increased catabolism of this particle impairing reverse cholesterol transport.[6,8] The degree of reduction is dependent on the degree of hypertriglyceridemia as well as other factors such as obesity, medications, smoking, and diabetes treatment.

If the lipid profile fails to normalize after adequate treatment of diabetes is instituted and normoglycemia is attained, an underlying genetic hyperlipidemia or another secondary cause should be sought and treated. The American Diabetes Association and other lipid experts emphasize reduction of LDL when elevated, as the first priority in treating diabetic dyslipidemia. The target LDL cholesterol for Type 2 diabetes is ≤100 mg/dL – the same as in patients with overt vascular disease. It is reasonable to assume that middle-aged or older Type 2 diabetics have underlying vascular disease, even in the absence of any clinical signs and symptoms.

DRUGS

Many drugs influence lipid levels in potentially adverse ways and may affect cardiovascular risk; details of drug-induced lipid changes have been the subject of review.[9] If the lipid abnormality cannot be reversed by switching the culprit drug, then the drug-induced dyslipidemia should be treated like a primary hyperlipidemia.

Alcohol

Alcoholic fatty liver and hyperlipidemia result from the interaction of ethanol and its oxidation products with hepatic lipid metabolism.[10] Alcohol commonly results in hypertriglyceridemia due to increased hepatic production and impaired removal of VLDL.[11] Moderate alcohol consumption results in increased levels of HDL and a lower total cholesterol/HDL ratio due to increased formation and decreased removal of HDL-C; this most likely explains some of the protective effects of alcohol on coronary artery disease. However, alcohol exerts little to no effect on LDL-C.

Antihypertensives

The effect of antihypertensive drugs on lipids has been studied extensively over the years. Indeed, a recent meta-analysis performed on 474 clinical trials has demonstrated the deleterious as well as beneficial effects of many antihypertensives on the lipid profile.[12]

Diuretics in most (but not all) studies have an adverse effect on the lipid profile.[12] While loop diuretics have not been well studied, in general thiazides and chlorthalidone increase cholesterol, LDL-C, and triglycerides without affecting HDL.[12] This effect is both dose-dependent and short-term in nature, such that after 1 year of treatment the lipid levels return to baseline.[13] The mechanism of these effects is thought to be due to increased alpha-adrenergic activity, which inhibits lipoprotein lipase activity and thus increases triglycerides and decreases HDL. Diuretics may also worsen insulin resistance, which is also associated with dyslipidemia.

The effect of beta-blockers on serum lipids depends on their pharmacological characteristics. Non-selective and β_1-selective beta-blockers have little effect on cholesterol, but increase triglycerides and decrease HDL.[12] Despite this effect they are protective in patients who have sustained a myocardial infarction (MI). Beta-blockers with intrinsic sympathomimetic activity (such as pindolol) seem to be more lipid neutral, and newer beta-blockers such as carvedilol (a combined non-selective beta- and alpha-1 blocker) have been shown to increase HDL and decrease triglycerides in diabetics.[14]

In contrast to both diuretics and beta-blockers, alpha-blockers have a beneficial effect on the lipid profile as they increase HDL and decrease LDL-C.[12] Despite these positive effects, there may not be any associated protection against cardiovascular disease as evidenced by the higher risk of congestive heart failure, stroke, and cardiovascular disease seen in the doxazsoszin arm of the ALLHAT study.[15] Clonidine, calcium-channel blockers, and angiotensin-converting enzyme (ACE) inhibitors are all lipid neutral.[12]

In subjects with both hyperlipidemia and hypertension, an alpha-blocker, ACE inhibitor or calcium-channel blocker may be the preferred initial therapy. Low-dose thiazides (12.5 mg) can be added without affecting the lipid profile adversely.

While beta-blockers can worsen hypertriglyceridemia, they have also been shown to reduce the risk of coronary events in the post-MI subject.[15]

Glucocorticoids

Several studies have evaluated the lipid effects of systemic glucocorticoids used for various inflammatory diseases. Steroid-treated patients with systemic lupus erythematosus for example, show an increase in triglycerides by as much as 44 percent, an increase in HDL by 10 percent, and an increase in LDL by up to 20 percent.[16] Other studies in subjects with rheumatoid arthritis and chronic obstructive pulmonary disease have shown similar results.[17] The mechanism of action of glucocorticoids on lipid metabolism has been shown to be related to decreased lipoprotein lipase activity.

Sex steroids

The effects of testosterone on the lipid profile are not clear. Most studies of men on replacement doses of testosterone show a decrease in HDL,[18] whereas men using anabolic agents can have dramatic reductions in HDL of up to 70 percent of baseline.[19,20] In some of these studies, this dramatic reduction in HDL was accompanied by an equally dramatic increase in LDL, by as much as 60 percent of baseline.[19] Several studies have shown that testosterone affects hepatic lipase activity; this results in catabolism of HDL and is the likely mechanism for the observed decrease in HDL.[20-22]

Most women at some point in their lives are exposed to exogenous estrogens, either in the form of oral contraceptives, hormone replacement for menopause, selective estrogen receptor modulators (SERMs), and/or phytoestrogens. Often, the estrogens are in combination with progestins, and therefore the lipid alterations can differ depending on dosage and formulation.

In general, synthetic estrogens such as ethinyl estradiol raise HDL by 20–38 percent, (particularly the HDL_2 sub-fraction), and sometimes can markedly increase triglyceride levels into the range associated with pancreatitis.[23,24] The excess triglycerides result from increases in a large VLDL particle that is not thought to be atherogenic as it is not metabolized to intermediate-density lipoprotein (IDL). Synthetic estrogens reduce lipoprotein (a) [Lp(a)] by 15–20 percent, total cholesterol by 10 percent, and LDL-C by up to 30 percent.[25] Slight attenuation of the above is seen with the natural estrogens, conjugated equine estrogen, and micronized estradiol. In contrast, transdermal estrogen has little effect on lipoproteins due to the absence of a first-pass effect through the liver where lipoprotein synthesis occurs;

hence, this approach should be used in dyslipidemic women with elevated triglycerides.

SERMs have specific tissue selective effects, as well as differential binding to the two known estrogen receptors, and can theoretically differ in terms of their effects on the lipid profile. Tamoxifen – a SERM with a mixed agonist-antagonist profile – is predominantly an estrogen agonist in the liver and can produce similar effects on the lipid profile as estrogen, including severe hypertriglyceridemia associated with pancreatitis.[28] Like estrogen, tamoxifen lowers LDL and has a variable effect on triglycerides;[26,27] HDL levels do not change. Raloxifene decreases LDL and has no effect on either triglycerides or HDL.

Oral contraceptives, depending on the type and amount of progestin that they contain, can be either lipid-favorable, lipid-neutral, or lipid-unfavorable.[29] The adverse effect of the progestin is proportional to its androgenicity. Norethindrone and norgestrel, being the most androgenic of the progestins, will lower HDL and increase LDL-C. Lipid-neutral progestins, which do not attenuate the favorable effect of estrogens, include gestodene, desogestrel, and norgestimate. Most low-dose 'triphasic' oral contraceptives have little to no significant effects on the lipid profile.

The phytoestrogens (e.g. daidzen and genistein) are found in soy and other food products, and may have the same effects on lipoproteins as exogenous estrogen.

Protease inhibitors

Lipid abnormalities are common in patients with HIV infection, and usually consist of hypocholesterolemia and moderate hypertriglyceridemia.[30] Protease inhibitor-based antiretroviral therapy has been associated with several metabolic complications,[31] including a syndrome of peripheral lipodystrophy (fat wasting of face, limbs and upper trunk), central adiposity, dorsocervical and supraclavicular fat pads, breast hypertrophy in women, hyperlipidemia, and insulin resistance,[32] as well as lipid abnormalities including hypercholesterolemia and sometimes severe hyper-triglyceridemia.[33–36] Ritonavir exhibits the most rapid and pronounced effect on cholesterol as well as triglyceride elevation.[31,34] All protease inhibitors have been reported to cause an increase in Lp(a).[34]

The mechanism by which protease inhibitors increase these lipid levels remains unknown. The significance of the alterations in lipid metabolism and their effect on the risks for pancreatitis and atherosclerosis in this population remain to be established, but it may be prudent to substitute one protease inhibitor for another in patients with protease inhibitor-associated hyperlipidemia. Guidelines for the treatment of dyslipidemia in patients with HIV are now available.[37]

HYPOTHYROIDISM

Untreated hypothyroidism has been associated with increased risk for atherosclerosis attributed in part to an accompanying hyperlipidemia. Hypothyroidism has been associated with virtually all common lipid abnormalities, although Type IIa is the most common lipid profile, seen in 56 percent of patients with primary hypo-thyroidism, and Type IIb is seen in 34 percent.[38] The primary mechanism for the hypercholesterolemia is explained by a decrease in cell surface LDL receptors, therefore decreasing LDL catabolism.[39] However, since thyroid hormone can decrease LPL activity, hypertriglyceridemia and abnormal remnant catabolism can also be seen.[40]

With restitution of the euthyroid state, the lipid profile improves significantly, especially in females.[38] When hypothyroidism coexists with an underlying genetic lipoprotein abnormality, marked exacerbation of the abnormal lipid profile can occur, but this will improve significantly with the institution of thyroid hormone replacement.[41] A recent analysis of 19 studies evaluating the effect of thyroid hormone replacement in patients with hypothyroidism demonstrated impressive reductions in total cholesterol levels of between 15 and 40 percent.[42]

The prevalence of both sub-clinical and overt hypothyroidism in patients with hypercholesterolemia has been demonstrated to be 4.4 percent and 2.8 percent, respectively.[43] Thus, all patients with hyperlipidemia should be screened for hypothyroidism prior to the institution of lipid-lowering therapy. If decreased thyroid function is documented, one should allow for 3–4 months of thyroid hormone replacement. If lipid levels are still elevated, then lipid-lowering therapy may be instituted.

NEPHROTIC SYNDROME

Nephrotic syndrome is recognized by the presence of proteinuria, lipiduria (mostly HDL), edema, hypoalbuminemia, and hypercholesterolemia, and is caused by a wide variety of systemic or primary renal diseases. One consequence, if untreated, may be accelerated atherosclerosis.

When hypoalbuminemia occurs, hepatic lipoprotein synthesis and clearance is altered, resulting in increased chylomicrons, VLDL, LDL, and Lp(a), but with little change in HDL concentration.[44,45] The degree of hypercholesterolemia is generally inversely proportional to the plasma albumin concentration as well as the plasma oncotic pressure, and can be improved transiently by albumin infusions.[46] In one study of 100 patients with nephrotic syndrome, 87 percent had total cholesterol levels >200 mg/dL, and 53 percent had levels >300 mg/dL.[47] In addition to changes in the hepatic synthesis of lipoproteins, removal of chylomicrons, VLDL and remnant particles is impaired[48,49] due to diminished LPL activity.[50]

Studies regarding the need for treatment are difficult to interpret, as many patients have remission of their nephrotic syndrome with treatment, and may not need lipid-lowering therapy in the short term. In patients with progressive end-stage renal disease, however, therapy is probably wise. There is evidence that the hyperlipidemia per se may in fact worsen renal function. LDL – and particularly oxidized LDL – has been shown in vitro to alter mesangial cell function and increase synthesis of extracellular matrix that may accelerate glomerulosclerosis.[51–55] Therefore, it is recommended that lipid-lowering therapy be instituted in those patients in whom the disease does not remit. The most widely used agents are the hexamethyl-glutaryl coenzyme A (HMG-CoA) reductase inhibitors, as it has been shown that the activity of this enzyme is increased in the nephrotic syndrome.[56]

RENAL DISEASE

Renal failure frequently causes alterations in lipoproteins, and thereby contributes to the high cardiovascular mortality seen in this population. Hypertriglyceridemia is the most common abnormality, especially in the pre-dialysis state.[56] The hyper-triglyceridemia is due to diminished clearance of VLDL and IDL and is accompanied by low HDL levels.

Alterations in the composition of the lipoproteins have also been described. Increased apolipoprotein C-III on triglyceride-rich lipoproteins is one of the earliest signs of dyslipoproteinemia in patients with declining renal function.[57] This alteration of apoprotein content impairs clearance of these triglyceride-rich particles, and leads to further accumulation. An increase in apoprotein B-containing lipoproteins may be an independent risk factor for the progression of renal disease, and consequently statin therapy has been proposed as a potential intervention to slow the rate of functional decline.[58] Renal transplant patients demonstrate similar disruptions in lipoproteins (see below), though some authors have reported predominantly hypercholesterolemia.[59]

The treatment of hypertriglyceridemia is generally only dietary in nature, as fibric acids have shown no long-term proven benefit and are associated with increased risk of rhabdomyolysis. In subjects with hypercholesterolemia, HMG-CoA reductase inhibitors can lower cholesterol levels safely.

TRANSPLANTATION

Renal transplantation can sometimes correct the abnormal lipid profile seen with renal failure and nephrosis. However, a significant number of patients have hypercholesterolemia and hypertriglyceridemia, with accumulation of remnant particles which can persist over many years. In addition, the immunosuppressant drugs used to prevent rejection can also cause hyperlipidemia.

Several studies have suggested that atherogenic changes in the lipid profile are worse with certain immunosuppressants such as cyclosporine, when compared to tacrolimus.[60–62] Glucocorticoids can cause both hypercholesterolemia and hyper-triglyceridemia, and cyclosporine can increase LDL-C (see above). Patients who develop chronic rejection frequently have hyperlipidemia, particularly hyper-triglyceridemia.[63]

Most studies have shown that renal transplant patients suffer a high morbidity and mortality due to premature cardiovascular disease. Therefore, aggressive treatment of the hyperlipidemia is recommended. Unfortunately, the use of high-dose statins is limited in this group due to the predisposition of precipitating rhabdomyolysis in the setting of cyclosporine use. To date, no trial has demonstrated improved cardiovascular outcomes with lipid-lowering therapy in the setting of renal transplantation. The ongoing ALERT trial (Assessment of Lescol in Renal

Transplantation) is due to report its findings in 2003.[64] Current recommendations regarding transplant-related hyperlipidemia include avoidance of obesity, and selection of the optimal immunosuppressive treatment, and the use (if possible) of agents that are lipid neutral.[65]

LIVER DISEASE

The liver plays a major role in the synthesis, storage, and metabolism of lipoproteins. Therefore, hepatic dysfunction can cause a variety of profound disturbances in the lipoprotein system as a result of the disturbed biosynthesis and/or impaired removal and metabolism of lipoprotein particles.

Both cholestasis and primary biliary cirrhosis are frequently associated with hypercholesterolemia and hypertriglyceridemia.[66] Triglyceride-rich remnants accumulate in plasma due to reduced plasma lipolytic activity and/or disturbed hepatic uptake. In addition, cholestasis causes a unique disturbance where a lipoprotein particle known as lipoprotein-X is produced from bile acids. Lipoprotein-X, a particle in the LDL density class, contains apoproteins C and D which are not found on the LDL particle. Lipoprotein-X may inhibit the hepatic apoprotein E receptor, thereby causing a marked inhibition of remnant particle uptake. When severely elevated (cholesterol >2000 mg/dL), lipoprotein X has been associated with hyperviscosity, but to date has not been associated with risk of atherosclerosis.[67]

Patients with primary biliary cirrhosis also exhibit low Lp(a) and elevated HDL-C levels.[68,69] These effects, combined with the unknown atherogenic potential of lipoprotein-X, may be responsible for the lack of atherogenic risk seen in this condition until now.

OBESITY

Most obese subjects are found to have hypertriglyceridemia accompanied by low HDL-C. Central obesity, in particular, has been noted to be associated with insulin resistance. Intra-abdominal fat has been implicated as the main fat store responsible for insulin resistance, as well as elevated levels of free fatty acids.[70] Consequently, the liver secretes Apo B-100 lipoproteins, and hepatic lipase is activated; this leads to the removal of cholesterol from LDL and HDL and results in the formation of small, dense particles. An atherogenic lipoprotein profile of hypertriglyceridemia – small dense LDL and decreased HDL_2 – is therefore characteristic of central obesity and insulin resistance.

SUMMARY

Secondary causes of hyperlipidemia are common, and are often forgotten or ignored as a potential source of intervention that might significantly improve lipid abnormalities. All patients with hyperlipidemia should be evaluated for some of the more common disorders discussed above, such as diabetes, hypothyroidism, liver and renal disorders, as well as for the use of certain medications that cause or exacerbate hyperlipidemia. A cost-effective approach to the laboratory evaluation useful for detecting secondary hyperlipidemia would include: thyroid-stimulating hormone, urinalysis, glucose, creatinine, and alkaline phosphatase. In addition, emphasis should be placed on treatment of the underlying disorder or consideration of stopping/changing possible culprit medications before lipid-lowering therapy is started.

REFERENCES

1. Garg A. Management of dyslipidemia in IDDM patients. *Diabetes Care* 1994; **17**: 224–34.
2. Sniderman AD, Scantlebury T, Cianflone K. Hypertriglyceridemic hyperapo B: the unappreciated atherogenic dyslipoproteinemia in type 2 diabetes mellitus. *Ann Intern Med* 2001; **135**: 447–59.
3. Kreisberg RA. Diabetic dyslipidemia. *Am J Cardiol* 1998; **82**: 67U–73U; discussion 85U–86U.
4. Betteridge DJ. Diabetic dyslipidemia. *Eur J Clin Invest* 1999; **29** (Suppl. 2): 12–16.
5. Fielding CJ, Reaven GM, Liu G, Fielding PE. Increased free cholesterol in plasma low and very low density lipoproteins in non-insulin-dependent diabetes mellitus: its role in the inhibition of cholesteryl ester transfer. *Proc Natl Acad Sci USA* 1984; **81**: 2512–16.
6. Abate N, Vega GL, Garg A, Grundy S. Abnormal distribution among lipoprotein fractions in normolipidemic patients with mild NIDDM. *Atherosclerosis* 1995; **118**: 111–22.
7. Wagner AM, Perez A, Calvo F, Bonet R, Castellvi A, Ordonez J. Apolipoprotein (B) identifies dyslipidemic phenotypes associated with cardiovascular risk in normocholesterolemic type 2 diabetic patients. *Diabetes Care* 1999; **22**: 812–17.
8. Golay A, Zech L, Shi M, Chiou YA, Reaven GM, Chen YD. High density lipoprotein (HDL) metabolism in non-insulin-dependent diabetes mellitus: measurement of HDL turnover using tritiated HDL. *J Clin Endocrinol Metab* 1987; **65**: 512–18.
9. Mantel-Teeuwisse AK, Kloosterman JME, Maitlan-van der Zee AH, et al. Drug-induced lipid changes: A review of the unintended effects of some commonly used drugs on serum lipid levels. *Drug Safety* 2001; **24**: 443–56.
10. Baraona E, Lieber CS. Alcohol and lipids. *Recent Dev Alcohol* 1998; **14**: 97–134.
11. Seidel D. Lipoproteins in liver disease. *J Clin Chem Clin Biochem* 1987; **25**: 541–51.
12. Kasiske BL, Ma JZ, Kalil RS, Louis, RA. Effects of antihypertensive therapy on serum lipids. *Ann Intern Med* 1995; **122**: 133–41.
13. Lakshman MR, Reda DJ, Materson BJ, et al. Diuretics and beta blockers do not have adverse effects at 1 year on plasma lipid and lipoprotein profiles in men with hypertension. *Arch Intern Med* 1999; **159**: 551–8.
14. ALLHAT Collaborative Research Group. Major cardiovascular events in hypertensive patients randomized to doxazosin vs. chlorthalidone: the antihypertensive and lipid-lowering treatment to prevent heart attack trial (ALLHAT). *JAMA* 2000; **283**: 1967–75.
15. Giugliano D, Acampora R, Marfella R, De Rosa N, Ziccardi P, Ragone R, De Angelis L, D'Onofrio F. Metabolic and cardiovascular effects of carvedilol and atenolol in non-insulin-dependent diabetes mellitus and hypertension. A randomized, controlled trial. *Ann Intern Med* 1997; **126**: 955–9.

16. Ettinger WH, Goldberg AP, Applebaum-Bowden D, *et al*. Dyslipoproteinemia in systemic lupus erythematosus: effect of corticosteroids. *Am J Med* 1987; **83**: 503–8.

17. El-Shaboury AH, Hayes TM. Hyperlipidemia in asthmatic patients receiving long-term steroid therapy. *Br Med J* 1973; **2**: 85–6.

18. Tan KC, Shiu SW, Pang RW, Kung AW. Effects of testosterone replacement on HDL subfractions and apolipoprotein A-1 containing lipoproteins. *Clin Endocrinol (Oxf.)* 1998; **48**: 187–94.

19. Hurley BF, Seals DR, Hagberg JM, Goldberg AC, Ostrove SM, Holloszy JO, Wiest WG, Goldberg AP. High density lipoprotein cholesterol in bodybuilders v. powerlifters: negative effects of androgen use. *JAMA* 1984; **252**: 507–13.

20. Kantor MA, Bianchini A, Bernier D, Sady SP, Thompson PD. Androgens reduce HDL2 cholesterol and increase hepatic triglyceride lipase activity. *Med Sci Sports Exerc* 1985; **17**: 462–5.

21. Haffner SM, Kushwaha RS, Foster DM, Applebaum-Bowden D, Hazzard WR. Studies on the metabolic mechanism of reduced high density lipoproteins during anabolic steroid therapy. *Metabolism* 1983; **32**: 413–20.

22. Sorva R, Kuusi T, Dunkel L, Taskinen MR. Effects of endogenous sex steroids on serum lipoproteins and postheparin plasma lipolytic enzymes. *J Clin Endocrinol Metab* 1988; **66**: 408–13.

23. Buckman MT, Johnson J, Ellis H, Srivastava L, Peake GT. Differential lipemia and proteinemic response to oral ethinyl estradiol and parenteral estradiol cypionate. *Metabolism* 1980; **29**: 803–5.

24. Ottosson UB, Carlstrom K, Hohansson BG, von Schoutz B. Estrogen induction of liver proteins and high density lipoprotein cholesterol: comparison between estradiol valerate and ethinyl estradiol. *Gynecol Obstet Invest* 1986; **22**: 198–205.

25. Henkin Y, Como JA. Secondary dyslipidemia: inadvertent effects of drugs in clinical practice. *JAMA* 1992; **267**: 961–8.

26. Colls BM, George PM. Severe hypertriglyceridaemia and hypercholesterolaemia associated with tamoxifen use. *Clin Oncol (R Coll Radiol)* 1998; **10**: 270–1.

27. Hozumi Y, Kawano M, Saito T, Miyata M. Effect of tamoxifen on serum lipid metabolism. *J Clin Endocrinol Metab* 1998; **83**: 1633–5.

28. Elisaf MS, Nakou K, Liamis G, Pavlidis NA. Tamoxifen-induced severe hypertriglyceridemia and pancreatitis. *Ann Oncol* 2000; **11**: 1067–9.

29. Godsland IF, Crook D, Simpson R, Proudler T, Felton C, Lees B, Anyaoku V, Devenport M, Wynn V. The effects of different formulations of oral contraceptive agents on lipid and carbohydrate metabolism. *N Engl J Med* 1990; **323**: 1375–81.

30. Grunfeld C, Kotler DP, Hamadeh R, Tierney A, Wang J, Pierson RN. Hypertriglyceridemia in the acquired immunodeficiency syndrome. *Am J Med* 1989; **86**: 27–31.

31. Jain RG, Furtine ES, Pedneault L, *et al*. Metabolic complications associated with antiretroviral therapy. *Antiviral Res* 2001; **51**: 151–77.

32. Carr A, Samaras K, Burton S, Law M, Freund J, Shisholm DJ, Cooper DA. A syndrome of peripheral lipodystrophy, hyperlipidaemia and insulin resistance in patients receiving HIV protease inhibitors. *AIDS* 1998; **12**: F51–8.

33. Echevarria KL, Hardin TC, Smith JA. Hyperlipidemia associated with protease inhibitor therapy. *Ann Pharmacother* 1999; **33**: 859–63.

34. Periard D, Telenti A, Sudre P, Cheseauz JJ, Halfon P, Reymond MJ, Marcovina SM, Glauser MP, Nicod P, Darioli R, Mooser V. Atherogenic dyslipidemia in HIV-infected individuals treated with protease inhibitors. The Swiss Cohort Study. *Circulation* 1999; **100**: 700–5.

35. Perry RC, Cushing HE, Deeg MA, Prince MJ. Ritonavir, triglycerides and pancreatitis. *Clin Infect Dis* 1999; **28**: 161–2.
36. Rakotoambinina B, Medioni J, Rabian C, *et al*. Lipodystrophic syndromes and hyperlipidemia in a cohort of HIV-infected patients receiving triple combination antiretroviral therapy with a protease inhibitor. *J Acq Immune Defic Syndr* 2001; **27**: 443–9.
37. Dube MP, Sprecher D, Henry WL, *et al*. Preliminary guidelines for the evaluation and management of dyslipidemia in adults infected with human immunodeficiency virus and receiving antiretroviral therapy: recommendations of the adult AIDS clinical trial group cardiovascular disease focus group. *Clin Infect Dis* 2000; **31**: 1216–24.
38. O'Brien T, Dinneen SF, O'Brien PC, Palumbo PJ. Hyperlipidemia in patients with primary and secondary hypothyroidism. *Mayo Clin Proc* 1993; **68**: 860–6.
39. Thompson GR, Soutar AK, Spengel FA, Jadhav A, Gavigan SJ, Myant NB. Defects of receptor mediated low density lipoprotein catabolism in homozygous familial hypercholesterolemia and hypothyroidism. *Proc Natl Acad Sci USA* 1981; **78**: 2591–5.
40. Pykalisto O, Goldberg A, Brunzell JD. Reversal of decreased human adipose tissue lipoprotein lipase and hypertriglyceridemia after treatment of hypothyroidism. *J Clin Endocrinol Metab* 1976; **43**: 591–600.
41. Pazos F, Alvarez JJ, Rubies-Pratt J, Varela C, Lasuncion MA. Long term thyroid replacement therapy and levels of lipoprotein(a) and other lipoproteins. *J Clin Endocrinol Metab* 1995; **80**: 862–6.
42. Tanis BC, Westendorp GJ, Smelt HM. Effect of thyroid substitution on hypercholesterolaemia in patients with subclinical hypothyroidism: a reanalysis of intervention studies. *Clin Endocrinol (Oxf.)* 1996; **44**: 643–9.
43. Tsimihodimos V, Bairaktari E, Tsallas C, *et al*. The incidence of thyroid function abnormalities in patients attending an outpatient lipid clinic. *Thyroid* 1999; **9**: 365–8.
44. Wheeler DC, Bernard DB. Lipid abnormalities in the nephrotic syndrome: causes, consequences and treatment. *Am J Kidney Dis* 1994; **23**: 331.
45. Kaysen GA, de Sain-van der Velden MGM. New insights into lipid metabolism in the nephrotic syndrome. *Kidney Int* 1999; **55** (Suppl.7): S18–21.
46. Baxter JH, Goodman HC, Allen JC. Effects of infusions of serum albumin on serum lipids and lipoproteins in nephrosis. *J Clin Invest* 1961; **49**: 490–8.
47. Radhakrishnan J, Appel AS, Valeri A, Appel GB. The nephrotic syndrome, lipids, and risk factors for cardiovascular disease. *Am J Kidney Dis* 1993; **22**: 135–42.
48. Furukawa S, Hirano T, Mamo J, Nagano S, Takahashi T. Catabolic defect of triglyceride is associated with abnormal very-low-density lipoproteins in experimental nephrosis. *Metabolism* 1990; **39**: 101–7.
49. Vaziri ND, Liang KH. Downregulation of hepatic LDL receptor expression in experimental nephrosis. *Kidney Int* 1996; **50**: 887–93.
50. Kashyap ML, Srivastava LS, Hynd BA, Brady D, Perisutti C, Glueck C, Gartside PS. Apoprotein CII and lipoprotein lipase in human nephrotic syndrome. *Atherosclerosis* 1980; **35**: 29–40.
51. Wheeler DC, Chana RS. Interactions between lipoproteins, glomerular cells, and matrix. *Miner Electrolyte Metab* 1993; **19**: 149–64.
52. Grone EF, Abboud HE, Hohne M, Walli AK, Grone HJ, Stuker D, Robenek H, Wieland E, Seidel D. Actions of lipoproteins in cultured human mesangial cells: modulation by mitogenic vasoconstrictors. *Am J Physiol* 1992; **263** (4 pt 2): F686–96.
53. Wasserman J, Santiago A, Rifici V, Holthofer H, Scharschmidt L, Epstein M, Schlondorff D. Interactions of low-density lipoprotein with rat mesangial cells. *Kidney Int* 1989; **35**: 1168–74.

54. Neugarten J, Schlondorff D. Lipoprotein interactions with glomerular cells and matrix. *Contemp Issues Nephrol* 1991; **24**: 173–206.
55. Moorhead JF, Chan MK, El-Nahas M, Varghese Z. Lipid nephrotoxicity in chronic progressive glomerular and tubulo-interstitial disease. *Lancet* 1982; **2**: 1309–11.
56. Appel GB, Blum CB, Chien S, Kunis CL, Appel AS. The hyperlipidemia of the nephrotic syndrome. *N Engl J Med* 1985; **312**: 1544–8.
57. Arnadottir M, Thysell H, Dallongeville J, Fruchart J, Nilsson-Ehle P. Evidence that reduced lipoprotein lipase activity is not a primary pathogenetic factor for hypertriglyceridemia in renal failure. *Kidney Int* 1995; **48**: 779–84.
58. Oda H, Keane WF. Recent advances in statins and the kidney. *Kidney Int* 1999; **71** (Suppl.): S2–5.
59. Ong CS, Pollock CA, Caterson RJ, Mahony JF, Waugh DA, Ibels LS. Hyperlipidemia in renal transplant recipients: natural history and response to treatment. *Medicine* 1994; **73**: 215–23.
60. Taylor DO, Barr ML, Radovancevic B, Renlund DG, Mentzer RM, Jr, Smart FW, Tolman DE, Frazier OH, Young JB, VanVeldhuisen P. A randomized, multicenter comparison of tacrolimus and cyclosporine immunosuppressive regimens in cardiac transplantation: decreased hyperlipidemia and hypertension with tacrolimus. *J Heart Transplant* 1999; **4**: 336–45.
61. Charco R, Cantarell C, Vargas V, Capdevila L, Lazaro JL, Hidalgo E, Murio E, Margarit C. Serum cholesterol changes in long-term survivors of liver transplantation: a comparison between cyclosporine and tacrolimus therapy. *Liver Transpl Surg* 1999; **5**: 204–8.
62. Kohnle M, Simmerman U, Lutkes P, *et al.* Conversion from cyclosporine A to tacrolimus after kidney transplantation due to hyperlipidemia. *Transpl Int* 2000; **13** (Suppl. 1): S345–8.
63. Guijarro C, Massy ZA, Kasiske BL. Clinical correlation between renal allograft failure and hyperlipidemia. *Kidney Int* 1995; **52**: S56–9.
64. Fellstrom B. Impact and management of hyperlipidemia posttransplantation. *Transplantation* 2000; **70** (11 Suppl.): SS51–7.
65. Holdaas H, Fellstrom B, Holme I, *et al.* Effects of fluvastatin on cardiac events in renal transplant patients: ALERT (Assessment of Lescol in Renal Transplantation) study design and baseline data. *J Cardiovasc Risk* 2001; **8**: 63–71.
66. Seidel D. Lipoproteins in liver disease. *J Clin Chem Clin Biochem* 1987; **25**: 541–51.
67. Rosenson, RS, Baker AL, Chow M, Hay RV. Hyperviscosity syndrome in a hypercholesterolemic patient with primary biliary cirrhosis. *Gastroenterology* 1990; **98** (5 Pt 1): 1351–7.
68. Crippin J, Lindor K, Jorgensen R, *et al.* Hypercholesterolemia and atherosclerosis in primary biliary cirrhosis: what is the risk? *Hepatology* 1992; **15**: 858–62.
69. Gregory WL, Game FL, Farrer M. Reduced serum lipoprotein(a) levels in patients with primary biliary cirrhosis. *Atherosclerosis* 1994; **105**: 43–50.
70. Brunzell JD, Hokanson JE. Dyslipidemia of central obesity and insulin resistance. *Diabetes Care* 1999; **22** (Suppl. 3): C10–13.

5

What to measure and when

ERNST J SCHAEFER, LEO J SEMAN AND JUDITH R McNAMARA

INTRODUCTION

It was only approximately 30 years ago that a high-risk cholesterol level was considered one that exceeded 300 mg/dL (7.8 mmol/L). Low-density lipoprotein (LDL) and high-density lipoprotein (HDL) cholesterol were not determined clinically, and triglycerides were rarely measured. Since the late 1970s, however, total cholesterol, triglyceride, and high-density lipoprotein-cholesterol (HDL-C) measurements have represented the standard lipoprotein profile, and this profile is still an important tool in the diagnosis of lipoprotein disorders.

NCEP RECOMMENDATIONS FOR LIPOPROTEIN TESTING

Current guidelines published by the Adult Treatment Panel of the National Cholesterol Education Program (NCEP) recommend dietary treatment for all adults over age 20 years if their serum low-density lipoprotein-cholesterol (LDL-C) values are ≥160 mg/dL (4.1 mmol/L), or ≥130 mg/dL (3.4 mmol/L) in the presence of two or more coronary heart disease (CHD) risk factors, or moderate CHD risk, or ≥100 mg/dL (2.6 mmol/L) in the presence of CHD, diabetes, or high CHD risk.[1,2] In addition, a decreased HDL-C level of <40 mg/dL (1.0 mmol/L) is a significant independent CHD risk factor, while an elevated level ≥60 mg/dL (1.55 mmol/L) is protective for CHD. After an adequate trial of a fat- and cholesterol-restricted diet (total fat ≤30% of calories, saturated fat <7%, and cholesterol <200 mg/day), and after ruling out secondary causes of hypercholesterolemia, especially thyroid, renal and liver diseases, persons with LDL-C values ≥190 mg/dL (4.9 mmol/L), or ≥160 mg/dL (4.1 mmol/L) in the presence of two or more CHD risk factors, or moderate CHD risk, or ≥130 mg/dL (3.4 mmol/L) in the presence of CHD, diabetes, or high CHD risk are candidates for pharmacological therapy with agents such as hydroxymethlyglutaryl-CoA (HMG-CoA) reductase inhibitors, anion-exchange resins, niacin, fibric acid derivatives, or a combination of these agents. The rationale for these guidelines is the association between increased LDL-C concentrations and premature CHD in prospective studies, and the fact that lowering LDL-C has been shown to reduce CHD risk prospectively.

According to the 2001 NCEP screening guidelines, screening for total cholesterol (TC), triglyceride (TG), and HDL-C after an overnight fast has been recommended for all adults over the age of 20 years. Serum or plasma TC and HDL-C concentrations can be measured in either the fasting or non-fasting state for screening purposes, but TG require a fasting measurement.[2] EDTA plasma values for TC are approximately 3 percent lower, and HDL-C levels are approximately 5 percent lower, than serum or heparin plasma values, and should be adjusted upward if EDTA is used. Compact analyzers using finger-stick specimens are available for TC, TG, and HDL-C.[3] Direct measurement of LDL-C can also be performed at screening, if available. It should be noted that non-fasting LDL-C and HDL-C will be physiologically slightly lower than comparable fasting samples due to transfer of cholesterol out of the LDL and HDL particles and into the triglyceride-rich lipoproteins, chylomicrons and very low-density lipoproteins (VLDL), post-prandially as they are synthesized.[4,5]

LDL-cholesterol

Prospective studies indicate that dietary treatment or a combination of dietary and drug therapy, which decreases LDL-C, can reduce subsequent CHD morbidity and mortality.[6-24] The results of several studies also indicate that aggressive reduction of LDL-C concentrations to <100 mg/dL (2.6 mmol/L) in patients with established CHD can stabilize existing coronary atherosclerosis, and possibly induce some regression.[11,25-35] Small angiographic changes appear to translate into large clinical benefits in CHD event reduction, consistent with plaque stabilization.[29,30,32] Because of these studies, consensus was reached on the use of medication to lower LDL-C concentrations.[36]

HDL cholesterol and triglycerides

While no definitive targets for TG-lowering or HDL-C-raising were established by ATP III, the panel suggested optimal levels for TG of <150 mg/dL (<1.70 mmol/L) and for HDL-C of >40 mg/dL (>1.0 mmol/L). Moreover, implicit in the panel report is the recommendation that after LDL-C targets are reached, one should strive to optimize both TG and HDL-C levels, especially in patients with CHD, diabetes, or high CHD risk.[2,37] A decreased level of HDL-C (<40 mg/dL or 1.0 mmol/L) has been shown to be an independent CHD risk factor, and increases in HDL-C concentrations were associated with a reduced CHD risk in both the Lipid Research Clinics – Coronary Primary Prevention Trial (LRC – CPPT)[6,7,38,39] and the Helsinki Heart Study.[18]

Recently the Veterans Administration HDL Intervention Trial (VA-HIT), a secondary prevention study of 2500 men, found a significant reduction in primary and secondary endpoints in men in whom HDL-C concentrations were increased while taking gemfibrozil, as compared with those taking placebo during a mean follow-up period of 5.1 years.[40] The men admitted into the study had established CHD, but had relatively normal LDL-C and TG levels; that is, LDL-C <140 mg/dL (3.6 mmol/L) and TG <300 mg/dL (3.4 mmol/L), and low HDL-C levels of <40 mg/dL (1.0 mmol/L) at baseline. The magnitude of change in HDL-C associated with CHD benefit was small, but significant. Importantly, the 7.5 percent increase in HDL-C, and 24.5 percent decrease in TG was associated with a 22 percent decrease in the incidence of coronary events. LDL-C values were not different between the placebo and gemfibrozil groups at baseline or during follow-up. A subsequent analysis of the data showed that the primary benefit was due to the rise in HDL-C levels.[41]

The contribution of increases in TG concentration to CHD risk has been controversial. TG have been shown to be an independent CHD risk factor in a meta-analysis,[42] especially in women, but this relationship has not been seen in most individual studies; an exception was a report from the Framingham Heart Study showing an independent association in women, but not in men.[43] TG are often used to calculate LDL-C concentration, using the formula of Friedewald et al. [(LDL-C = TC − HDL-C − TG/5) for mg/dL or (LDL-C = TC − HDL-C − TG/2.22) for mmol/L].[44] Triglyceride measurements are also important for the diagnosis and monitoring of individuals with severe hypertriglyceridemia. Borderline hyper-triglyceridemia (150–199 mg/dL; 1.70–2.25 mmol/L) is associated with decreased HDL-C levels, and is commonly found in diabetics and CHD patients. Severe hypertriglyceridemia (>1000 mg/dL; >11 mmol/L), although not associated with CHD, can result in pancreatitis; this is a life-threatening condition and is therefore important to ascertain and treat.

In both the Lipid Research Clinics Trial and the Helsinki Heart Study, it was shown that raising HDL-C concentration with medication was beneficial for CHD risk reduction along with LDL-C lowering, but no such data are available for TG-lowering.[6,7,17,18,38] Surprisingly, despite a 34 percent reduction in TG in the Helsinki Heart Study, no reduction in CHD risk reduction could be associated with this reduction.[18] For these reasons, previous NCEP Adult Treatment Panels focused on LDL-C concentrations. However, data from the LRC – CPPT, Helsinki Heart Study, and VA-HIT support the concept of raising HDL-C levels to over 40 mg/dL to reduce CHD risk.[18,38,41] Based on the VA-HIT data, this recommendation can certainly be made in CHD patients.[41]

PRE-ANALYTICAL ISSUES

When obtaining blood for lipoprotein measurements, whether from finger-stick or a venous blood draw, it is important for patients to be properly instructed in order to obtain reliable results. Patients should ideally be in a steady state in which they have not made major lifestyle changes during the month prior to the blood draw.

- Any dietary, medication, or exercise changes should be stabilized for at least 4 weeks before lipoprotein testing is performed.
- Biological variability is dependent on the individual and the assay to be measured. Some individuals are more sensitive to slight changes in their environment (diet, exercise, etc.) than other individuals. Because of this, the NCEP has recommended two measurements, to be made several weeks apart, before any definitive diagnosis is made. If there are substantial differences between the results, more measurements may be required.[45]
- If a fasting lipoprotein profile is desired, the patient should fast for at least 9 h, and preferably 12–14 h, after a low-fat meal and should abstain from alcoholic beverages for 24 h prior to the blood draw, as each can have a marked effect on TG concentrations.[45]
- If a non-fasting sample is desired, fasting is not necessary, but TG should not be determined.
- Since vitamin C intake can affect lipid results by interfering with the enzymatic analytical reaction, blood samples should not be drawn within 4 h of vitamin C ingestion.
- Because lipid concentrations can change with body position, the standard blood-drawing procedures recommend sitting for a 5-min interval prior to the blood draw. A supine position, sometimes necessitated for in-hospital patients, will result in lower values than would be obtained in the seated position.[45] Cholesterol concentrations will be approximately 10 percent higher when standing than when prone, TG, approximately 12 percent higher, and HDL-C approximately 7 percent higher.[46] Although it can take approximately 30 min for complete equilibration when changing position, in usual practice, sitting quietly for 5 min before blood drawing accounts for the majority of the hemodynamic changes, and has become 'standard procedure.'
- Capillary blood has more potential for variability than venous blood, but is often used for screening purposes. Finger-sticks that provide a good flow of blood without 'milking', however, have been shown to provide reliable results.[47] Correct technique is important.
- Another effect on lipid concentrations is stress – both physiological (from interventional procedures and/or illness) and psychological (from worries about health status, impending procedures, and/or pain) – and these will lower both TC and HDL-C levels. Acute phase phenomena, as are seen in acute myocardial infarction, also depress cholesterol levels.[48,49] Viral infections can also significantly reduce TC and HDL-C concentrations, and blood draws should be rescheduled if possible. It is usually not necessary to determine lipid/lipoprotein concentrations in hospital when both physiological and psychological stress levels are likely to be

elevated; these analyses are better determined on an outpatient basis whenever possible.

LABORATORY ISSUES

Precision and accuracy

The NCEP Laboratory Standardization Panel and its successor, the NCEP Working Group on Lipoprotein Measurement, established precision and accuracy guidelines for laboratories for the purpose of assuring reliable and commutable lipid and lipoprotein results among laboratories, physician offices, and screening clinics.[50–53]

LDL-C: calculation or measurement

Today, LDL-C and HDL-C are considered to be the most important modifiable indicators of CHD risk, along with smoking, hypertension, and elevated serum glucose levels. It is therefore important that laboratory assessment of these analytes be precise and accurate. The formula commonly used to calculate LDL-C is: LDL-C = TC − HDL-C − TG/5, when values are in mg/dL (or TG/2.22 when values are in mmol/L),[44] but there are limitations to its use. It has been documented that this formula cannot be used for values from serum or plasma drawn from non-fasting individuals or from those whose TG values are >400 mg/dL (4.5 mmol/L). However, considerable variability in calculated LDL-C concentrations also exists when TG values are 200–400 mg/dL (2.3–4.5 mmol/L).[54] Data from our laboratory indicate that about 5 percent of the population has fasting TG values >400 mg/dL (4.5 mmol/L), but an additional 12 percent have TG levels in the range of 200–400 mg/dL. In the >400 mg/dL concentration range, approximately 75 percent of results are inaccurate by >10 percent in comparison with ultracentrifugation, but even in the 200–400 mg/dL range, >30 percent of results are inaccurate from 200 to 300 mg/dL, and >40 percent are inaccurate in the range of 300–400 mg/dL.

The Friedewald equation, in its use of TG/5, relies on two assumptions: (i) that all serum TG resides in VLDL; and (ii) that all VLDL contain 20 percent of their mass as cholesterol. The first assumption, while not totally correct, is reasonable since the majority of serum TG is found in VLDL when samples are relatively normo-triglyceridemic and are obtained in the truly fasting state (ideally, 12–14 h after a low-fat meal, with no alcoholic intake for 24 h). Only small amounts are carried in LDL and HDL. Significant quantities can be carried in chylomicrons in post-prandial and severely hypertriglyceridemic samples, however, and in intermediate-density lipoprotein (IDL) in the case of patients with Type III hyperlipoproteinemia. The second assumption is also very reliable when TG are fasting and relatively low (<250 mg/dL or <2.8 mmol/L). When TG are elevated, however, there are more likely to be particles present with abnormal composition, which may have a much higher proportion of cholesterol, such as in individuals with Type III hyperlipoproteinemia

(>30% of mass as cholesterol), or a much lower proportion, as in the case of non-fasting samples where chylomicrons are present (<10% of mass as cholesterol). The end result is that the formula does not provide accurate results when the composition of particles is abnormal. A reasonable solution is to use the Friedewald equation when samples are from fasting subjects and TG are below 250 mg/dL (2.8 mmol/L), but to use one of the direct LDL-C assays when either of those two conditions is lacking.

Even within the confines of precision and accuracy limits set by the NCEP Laboratory Standardization Panel and the Working Group on Lipoprotein Measurement for TC, LDL-C, HDL-C, and TG, it is possible for LDL-C concentrations, when estimated by the Friedewald formula, to be outside recommended limits. The NCEP Working Group on Lipoprotein Measurement, therefore, recommended the development of direct methods for measuring LDL-C.[50] The first direct LDL-C assay to be developed was designed to immunoprecipitate chylomicrons, VLDL, and HDL from serum or plasma, leaving LDL behind, and then to measure the LDL-C in the filtrate by automated enzymatic techniques. This assay was evaluated in multiple studies and found to correlate very highly with LDL-C measured following ultracentrifugation ($r = 0.88$ to 0.98) based on analyses of serum samples obtained from subjects with TG concentrations up to 4000 mg/dL (45 mmol/L).[55–57]. Within-run coefficients of variation (CVs) ranged from 1.2 to 3.8 percent, and between-run CVs ranged from 1.2 to 5.1 percent. Moreover, it was documented that this assay gave accurate and reliable results on non-fasting as well as fasting serum, and that it could be used for samples with very elevated TG levels.[55,57] It could not, however, be used with samples that had been previously frozen.[55] A second generation of 'homogeneous' assays has subsequently come to market, generally based on customized detergents as the basis for LDL isolation.[58] Homogeneous assays for HDL-C measurement have also been developed.[59] In general, these assays have the advantages of not requiring an initial precipitation step and of being able to be used for measurement in previously frozen samples. A disadvantage appears to be a limitation in the TG concentration range, such that samples with TG >~1000 mg/dL (11 mmol/L) provide less accurate values.

One major advantage of assays that actually measure LDL-C (reference and direct methods, alike) is the ability to assay non-fasting samples.[55,57] This fact makes it possible to add LDL-C measurements to screening panels. It should be borne in mind, however, that LDL-C concentrations measured in the post-prandial state will, in general, be slightly lower than comparable fasting samples, regardless of the method used, due to physiological changes.[11] The decreases are moderate, generally <3–5 percent, but may be as high as ~8 percent at the time of peak post-prandial triglyceridemia after a very high fat meal. The magnitude of LDL-C decrease will vary with the size and fat content of the meal, with the length of time following the meal, and with the metabolic efficiency of the individual. Decreases in the cholesterol content of LDL, and also of HDL, are due to transfer of cholesterol ester out of these particles and into newly synthesized chylomicrons and VLDL. While the serum concentration decreases are small, they should be kept in mind when interpreting borderline results.

OTHER ASSAYS AND THEIR UTILITY

Apolipoproteins A–I and B

Apolipoprotein (apo) A-I is the major protein of HDL; apo B is the major protein of LDL and VLDL, and as such they correlate highly with HDL-C and LDL-C, respectively. Apo A-I and apo B are commonly measured in research laboratories and in some clinical laboratories in addition to LDL-C and HDL-C. Measurement of both the lipid and protein moieties can provide more complete lipoprotein information than either the cholesterol or the protein alone, but in a clinical setting there is not enough extra information garnered for most individuals to support the additional costs of measuring both. Approximately the same amount of CHD risk information can be gained by measuring LDL-C and HDL-C *or* by measuring apo B and apo A-I. In the United States, however – where lipoprotein risk has traditionally been assessed by the use of lipid measurements – apolipoprotein measurements have not been recommended for routine use.

In some studies, decreased apo A-I levels and elevated apo B levels were reported to be superior to LDL-C and HDL-C concentrations as markers for CHD,[60–64] but these were all case-control studies. Apo A-I and apo B concentrations appear to be less affected by dietary modification and the use of adrenergic blocking agents than are TG, LDL-C, and HDL-C concentrations. Most CHD patients have modified their diet and are often on beta-blockers, and these represent confounders in such case-control studies.[65] Moreover, while several prospective studies have assessed the utility of apo A-I and apo B versus LDL-C and HDL-C concentrations as CHD markers, none has documented that apos added significant additional information about CHD risk.[66–72] Standardization for apo A-I and apo B is now available,[73–76] but apo A-I and apo B do not appear to provide significant additional clinical information. More data from large-scale prospective studies are required, however, before definitive conclusions can be reached.

Lipoprotein (a)

Elevated levels of lipoprotein(a) [Lp(a)] have been associated with increased risk of CHD in most studies,[77–93] although not all prospective studies have confirmed the association.[94,95] Lp(a) particles are synthesized in the liver, and consist of LDL particles with an extra apolipoprotein [called apo(a)] which is linked by a disulfide bond to apo B-100.[96,97] Apo(a) is heterogeneous in length due to differing numbers of repeating peptide sequences called kringles. Molecular weights range from approximately 185 kDa to 650 kDa, and protein length is genetically determined.[97,98]

The plasma concentration of Lp(a) is inversely related to the apo(a) isoform length, such that longer peptide chains are associated with lower plasma concentrations, and their density range (1.050–1.15 g/mL) overlaps the LDL and HDL density ranges.[97] On agarose gel electrophoresis, Lp(a) migrates in the pre-beta range, and was originally identified as sinking pre-beta lipoprotein.[96] In order to observe Lp(a) by agarose electrophoresis, however, it is necessary to perform ultracentrifugation first to isolate the 1.006 kg/L infranate. If whole plasma is applied to the gel, visualization of Lp(a) is obscured by the presence of VLDL, which also have pre-beta mobility. Apo(a) also has >75 percent homology with plasminogen,[100] and is thought to compete with plasminogen for fibrin binding sites, thereby interfering with fibrinolysis.[101–104]

Measurement of Lp(a) can be performed either by measurement of apo(a) protein concentration, which is then converted to an estimate of total Lp(a) particle mass (sum of the molar concentrations of the protein, cholesterol, triglyceride, and phospholipid that comprise the particles),[105] or by measurement of Lp(a) cholesterol concentration,[83,106] as is done for measurement of LDL and HDL concentration. Protein and cholesterol each account for approximately 30 percent of Lp(a) mass. Mass assays involving immunological separation of apo(a) use specific epitopes to avoid regions homologous to plasminogen and regions subject to kringle IV, type 2 sequences, which are the peptides that account for the size heterogeneity. The protein is then quantitated by enzyme-linked immunosorbent assay (ELISA), enzyme immunoassay (EIA), nephelometric, or turbidometric assays. For the Lp(a) cholesterol assay, Lp(a) are bound to lectin, taking advantage of their high degree of glycosylation. After eluting Lp(a) from the column, the cholesterol is measured. Standardization procedures and materials are currently being evaluated through the International Federation of Clinical Chemistry (IFCC) and the National Institutes of Health (NIH). Reference materials will be used by manufacturers to set calibrator concentrations in the same way that reference materials developed for apos A-I and B are used.

Lp(a) concentrations are unevenly distributed in Caucasian populations, with most individuals having very low concentrations. For example, in the third offspring examination of the Framingham Heart Study, the mean total mass concentration was approximately 15 mg/dL, whereas the median value was only 8 mg/dL.[107] Concentrations in some individuals can exceed 100 mg/dL, and can occasionally be found as high as 200–300 mg/dL. African Americans demonstrate a more Gaussian distribution of Lp(a) values than Caucasians, however, with a more elevated median level. In the CARDIA study, the median value for African Americans was three times higher than that for Caucasians.[108] It is not yet clear, however, whether the more elevated levels observed in the Black population confer greater CHD risk.[109–111] In general, however, an Lp(a) total mass concentration >30 mg/dL is considered elevated; the corresponding Lp(a) cholesterol cut-off point is 10 mg/dL.[112]

Despite the similarity between Lp(a) and LDL, most LDL-lowering drugs have little or no effect on Lp(a) concentrations. The only agents that have been shown to significantly decrease Lp(a) levels are niacin and estrogen replacement preparations for postmenopausal women. Prospective studies generally confirm the atherogenicity of Lp(a). Treatment with niacin in such patients with CHD can be recommended, since niacin has been shown to reduce CHD in unselected CHD patients.[112–114] Knowledge of an elevated Lp(a) level can also be used as an indication of the need to be particularly assertive in normalizing other modifiable CHD risk factors.

Triglyceride-rich lipoprotein remnants

While many CHD patients present with moderately elevated TG, independent associations between TG and CHD have been inconsistent.[115–118] Reasons for lack of association in many studies are probably related to biological variability and the compositional heterogeneity within TG-rich lipoproteins (TRL) that causes difficulty with the Friedewald calculation. TRL include chylomicrons, chylomicron remnants, VLDL, and VLDL remnants. Proposed mechanisms of action which may be involved include interference with vasorelaxation[119] and subendothelial accumulation of chylomicron remnants.[120,121]

Chylomicrons synthesized in the intestine after a meal rapidly undergo lipolysis via the action of the enzyme, lipoprotein lipase (LPL). During this process they lose much of their triglyceride and apo C, and gain cholesteryl ester and apo E via the action of cholesteryl ester transfer protein (CETP), resulting in what are then known as chylomicron remnants.[122] Chylomicron remnants contain apo B-48 as their major protein constituent, are enriched in apo E, as compared to nascent chylomicrons, and are eventually removed by the liver through a receptor-mediated process.

VLDL, another species of TRL, are synthesized in the liver, rather than the intestine, and contain apo B-100 in place of apo B-48. As with chylomicrons, VLDL have a hydrated density of <1.006 kg/L and are heterogeneous in size. Newly secreted VLDL also undergo lipolysis by LPL, losing much of their triglyceride and apo C, and gaining cholesteryl esters and apo E. Following lipolysis they are known as VLDL remnants, and are relatively apo E-enriched. The main compositional difference between VLDL remnants and chylomicron remnants is the presence of apo B-100, rather than apo B-48 as the major protein, and the relative TG concentration. VLDL remnants can undergo further metabolism to become IDL (density 1.006–1.019 kg/L), another form of TRL remnant which are even more cholesterol-enriched and TG-poor, but still contain apo E. Finally, after further hydrolysis and removal of apo E, LDL (density 1.019–1.063 kg/L) are formed. Alternatively, VLDL remnants can be removed from the circulation directly by the liver. Both chylomicron and VLDL remnants are thought to be atherogenic.[119–127]

Separation of remnant lipoproteins has always been very difficult because of overlapping size, density and composition among the native and remnant forms of TRL. Traditionally, remnants have been separated using ultracentrifugation and column separation techniques, which have not been suitable for large-scale studies. The ability to separate remnants, however, could possibly allow direct quantitation of the specific atherogenic subspecies within TRL; that is, remnants, without analyzing newly formed TRL which may not be atherogenic. Studies have shown that remnants can remain in circulation for extended periods of time post-prandially, even in individuals with normal fasting TG concentrations.[4,5,121,128–131]

An immunologically based assay has recently been developed, that allows isolation of a sub-set of TRL that are enriched in apo E, and display classical remnant-like characteristics.[132–134] Isolation is based on removal of apo A-I-containing particles (HDL) with an anti-apo A-I monoclonal antibody and most apo B-containing particles (primarily LDL and nascent VLDL), with a specific monoclonal antibody to apo B (JI-H), that does not recognize partially hydrolyzed, apo E-enriched lipoprotein remnants.[131–133] Unbound remnants remain in the supernate. Reference ranges have been generated for these remnant-like particles (RLP) in two populations,[135,136] and studies examining the relationship between RLP and cardiovascular disease (CVD) indicate an association,[125,127,137–139] although no large prospective studies have yet been completed.

Other areas where the RLP assay may eventually be of use to clinical laboratories is for risk assessment in diabetes,[140] and in the diagnosis of individuals with Type III hyperlipoproteinemia, or dysbetalipoproteinemia,[141,142] who are also at high risk for developing CVD. Diagnosis of Type III hyperlipoproteinemia currently requires ultracentrifugation to allow calculation of the VLDL-C to TG ratio (>0.3 in Type III patients) and to document the presence of beta-VLDL on agarose electrophoresis, and apo E phenotyping or genotyping to document an apo E 2/2 phenotype. Because of these requirements, many Type III patients are not identified and are categorized as combined hyperlipoproteinemia. Use of the ratio of RLP-C to TG could replace the VLDL-C to TG ratio, thereby eliminating the need for ultracentrifugation. Type III patients generally have elevated RLP-C concentrations (at or above the 75th percentile of the population) and RLP-C to TG ratios of >0.10.[142] In our view, elevated RLP-C concentrations can be effectively lowered with some HMG-CoA reductase inhibitors, such as atorvastatin.[143]

HOMOCYSTEINE

Homocysteinurias represent a class of inborn errors of metabolism that affect metabolism of sulfur-containing amino acids and result in extremely elevated plasma and urinary levels of homocysteine.[144] Untreated individuals with this defect frequently develop CVD by their teenage years and as early as infancy. It was therefore hypothesized that individuals with more moderate increases in homocysteine might also be at some increased level of CVD risk.[145,146] Most, but not all, studies have confirmed this concept.[147–156] The metabolic pathway involved in the synthesis and catabolism of homocysteine contains several enzymes which have the potential if defective or inactive to interfere with homocysteine metabolism and to result in its elevation. These enzymes include cystathionine beta-synthase, methylenetetrahydrofolate reductase, and N-5-methylenetetrahydrofolate:homocysteine methyltransferase.[156] Elevated plasma homocysteine levels have been associated with oxidative cell damage, vasoconstriction, vascular smooth muscle proliferation, and hypercoagulability,[157–159] all of which are potential mechanisms for the association of homocysteine with CVD risk.

Distribution of homocysteine levels in the population varies by age, gender, and ethnicity.[160,161] The elderly tend to have a lower dietary intake of B vitamins and have higher homocysteine concentrations as a result.[162–164] Other populations at increased risk of having hyperhomocysteinemia are diabetics[152–165] and patients with renal disease, as the kidney is the site of trans-sulfuration enzymes.[166,167]

For many individuals with increased concentrations of homocysteine, treatment is easily accomplished through supplementary intake of folate, B_6, and B_{12} vitamins.[165,168,169] Recent fortification of the United States grain supply with folate for the purpose of reducing the incidence of neural tube defect in fetuses is, as a secondary effect, reducing levels of homocysteine in the general population.[168,169] Whether this reduction will translate into a reduction in cardiac and vascular events will await future evaluation. Existing evidence gained from studies where homocysteine levels have been reduced would lead to the prediction that there will be a reduction in events.[150]

Laboratory analysis of homocysteine has generally been performed using high-performance liquid chromatography methodology, which makes this approach inaccessible to most clinical laboratories. With the positive association found in studies evaluating homocysteine as a CVD risk factor, however, new methods have started to be developed that are more useful in a clinical chemistry laboratory environment. We are now, therefore, beginning to see methodologies, such as immunoassays, that are more suitable to clinical laboratories[170,171] EDTA or heparin anticoagulants are generally preferred; plasma should be drawn in the fasting state, separated, and analyzed immediately or stored at −70°C, where it is stable for extended periods of time.

Issues important to the clinical laboratory measurement of homocysteine involve more than just measurement technology, however. One issue is the lack of standardization, and therefore the potential difficulty in comparing results among methods.[172]

There is also the issue of whether homocysteine levels will be requested frequently enough to make a homocysteine assay worth putting in place. Since homocysteine levels are decreased so easily in most individuals by vitamin supplementation, many physicians may elect to bypass measurement and go directly to supplementation. There are two problems with that approach, however: (i) supplementation with folate alone will mask, but not resolve, symptoms of pernicious anemia[164]; and (ii) defects in the thermolabile methylenetetrahydrofolate reductase enzyme will require greater levels of folate supplementation than would be required to normalize most increases in homocysteine.[173] This defect represents a common mutation found in individuals with elevated homocysteine concentrations, indicating that both initial and follow-up homocysteine concentrations should be measured.

LIPOPROTEIN SUB-FRACTIONATION AND SIZING

Plasma lipoproteins can differ significantly in size as determined by gradient gel electrophoresis. As many as eight different sizes of LDL particles occur in plasma, with most subjects having one major band and two or three adjacent satellite bands.[174,175] Mean LDL particle size is significantly larger in women than in men, and is heavily influenced by plasma TG levels.[174,176] Subjects with severe hyper-triglyceridemia have the smallest LDL particles, and subjects who lower their TG levels with weight loss, exercise, or TG-lowering medication will significantly increase their LDL particle size.[177] LDL particle size is not very heritable.[178,179]

Significant interest in LDL particle size was generated by the report that it was significantly smaller in CHD patients than in controls.[180] Austin et al. have divided LDL particle size into pattern A (large particles) and pattern B (small particles), and have reported that a high percentage of CHD patients have pattern B LDL.[180] CHD patients actually have LDL particles that are in the intermediate size range, and are enriched in cholesterol ester, and these types of LDL particles are associated with the highest levels of LDL-C.[175,177,181]

A new method of lipoprotein assessment by nuclear magnetic resonance (NMR) appears promising, and reports the TG content of one chylomicron fraction and six

VLDL fractions, along with the cholesterol content in one IDL fraction, three LDL fractions, and five HDL fractions. The method does not measure the lipids directly, and concentrations are relative. However, the patterns detected are of interest, and CHD patients have increases in the VLDL and small and medium LDL fractions, and decreases in the large HDL fractions.[182]

Most – but not all – current data indicate that LDL particle size does not add significant information about CHD risk, above and beyond that provided by previously mentioned lipid assays.[181,183,184] Moreover, LDL size measurements have not been standardized, and no large-scale prospective data are as yet available. Therefore, its routine measurement cannot be recommended at the present time.

C-REACTIVE PROTEIN

C-reactive protein (CRP) has been used as a marker of inflammation for many years, and is associated with 10-fold increases in concentration over baseline levels during an acute inflammatory event. These levels fall quickly back to normal levels when the inflammation has been eliminated.

Inflammation is also involved in the atherosclerotic process and therefore, the effectiveness of using inflammatory markers to predict future CVD events is of interest. CRP has been positively associated with CVD risk in most studies, independent of lipoprotein abnormalities.[185–190] It has also been shown to have a possible synergistic association with cholesterol[190] and insulin resistance.[191] Agents shown to reduce CRP levels include aspirin[190] and statin therapy.[192]

The association with atherosclerosis however represents a very low, but chronic, level of inflammation. The differences in CRP concentration between low and high levels of CVD risk are quite small, and concentrations associated with high risk actually fall within what is generally considered to be the upper level of normal range.[193] Sensitive assays for CRP are therefore necessary to evaluate these small differences between high and low risk. High-sensitivity assays (hsCRP) were developed for the studies that evaluated this marker for CVD risk, and others have since become commercially available for clinical laboratory use.[193–195]

CONCLUSION

This chapter is designed to provide an overview of the diagnosis and treatment of lipoprotein disorders and NCEP guidelines for therapy. Current diagnostic tests that are recommended include serum TC, TG, HDL-C, and calculated LDL-C in the fasting state. If fasting TG values are $\geq$250 mg/dL (2.8 mmol/L), then LDL-C should be measured using a direct assay, for greater accuracy. The routine measurement of apo A-I, apo B, or LDL size can not be recommended because of a lack of prospective data documenting that these assays provide significant additional information about CHD risk prediction. Lp(a) is an important addition to lipoprotein assessment, as it provides significant additional information about CHD risk, and can readily be measured. CRP may also become an important marker for risk, independent of the lipoprotein markers. In our view, in future the direct measurement of LDL-C, HDL-C – and perhaps also of RLP, along with serum TG and Lp(a) – will become standard practice in lipoprotein assessment. Moreover, researchers are actively developing methodologies that will eliminate pre-analytical steps, for increased precision, accuracy, and throughput.

REFERENCES

1. The Expert Panel. Report of the National Cholesterol Education Program Expert Panel on Detection, Evaluation, and Treatment of High Blood Cholesterol in Adults. *Arch Intern Med* 1988; **148**: 36–69.
2. Expert Panel on Detection, Evaluation, and Treatment of High Blood Cholesterol in Adults. Executive summary of the third report of the National Cholesterol Education Program (NCEP) Expert Panel on Detection, Evaluation, and Treatment of High Blood Cholesterol in Adults (Adult Treatment Panel III). *JAMA* 2001; **285**: 2486–97.
3. Kaufman HW, McNamara JR, Anderson KM, Wilson PWF, Schaefer EJ. How reliably can compact chemistry analyzers measure lipids? *JAMA* 1990; **263**: 1245–9.
4. Cohn JS, McNamara JR, Cohn SD, Ordovas JM, Schaefer EJ. Postprandial plasma lipoprotein changes in human subjects of different ages. *J Lipid Res* 1988; **29**: 469–79.
5. Cohn JS, McNamara JR, Schaefer EJ. Lipoprotein cholesterol concentrations in the plasma of human subjects as measured in the fed and fasted states. *Clin Chem* 1988; **34**: 2456–9.
6. The Lipid Research Clinics Program. The Lipid Research Clinics Coronary Primary Prevention Trial. I. Reduction in incidence of coronary heart disease. *JAMA* 1984; **251**: 351–64.
7. The Lipid Research Clinics Program. The Lipid Research Clinics Coronary Primary Prevention Trial. II. The relationship of reduction in incidence of coronary heart disease to cholesterol lowering. *JAMA* 1984; **251**: 365–74.
8. Dayton S, Pearce ML, Hashimoto S, Dixon WJ, Tomiyasu U. A controlled clinical trial of a diet high in unsaturated fat in preventing complications of atherosclerosis. *Circulation* 1969; **40** (Suppl. II): 11–63.
9. Hjermann I, Holme I, Byre KV, Leren P. Effect of diet and smoking intervention on the incidence of coronary heart disease. *Lancet* 1981; **2**: 1303–10.
10. Holme I, Hjermann I, Helgelend A, Leren P. The Oslo Study: diet and anti-smoking advice: additional results from a 5 year primary prevention trial in middle aged men. *Prev Med* 1985; **14**: 279–92.
11. Miettinen M, Karvonen MJ, Turpeinen O, Elosuo R, Paavilainen F. Effect of cholesterol lowering diet on mortality from coronary heart disease and other causes. A twelve year clinical trial in men and women. *Lancet* 1972; **2**: 835–8.
12. Ornish D, Brown SK, Scherwitz LW, *et al*. Can life-style changes reverse coronary heart disease? *Lancet* 1990; **326**: 129–33.
13. Leren P. The effect of plasma cholesterol lowering diet in male survivors of myocardial infarction. *Acta Med Scand* 1966; **466** (Suppl.): 92–116.
14. de Lorgeril M, Renaud S, Mamelle N, *et al*. Mediterranean alpha-linolenic acid-rich diet in secondary prevention of coronary heart disease. *Lancet* 1994; **343**: 1454–9.
15. Canner PL, Berge KG, Wenger NK, *et al*. Fifteen-year mortality in Coronary Drug Project patients: long-term benefit with niacin. *J Am Coll Cardiol* 1986; **8**: 1245–55.

16. Carlson LA, Rosenhamer G. Reduction of mortality in the Stockholm Ischemic Heart Disease Study by combined treatment with clofibrate and nicotinic acid. *Acta Med Scand* 1988; **223**: 405–18.

17. Frick MH, Elo O, Haapa K, *et al.* Helsinki Heart Study: primary prevention trial with gemfibrozil in middle-aged men with dyslipidemia. *N Engl J Med* 1987; **317**: 1237–45.

18. Manninen V, Elo O, Frick MH, *et al.* Lipid alterations and decline in the incidence of coronary heart disease in the Helsinki Heart Study. *JAMA* 1988; **260**: 641–51.

19. Manninen V, Tenkanen L, Koskinen P, *et al.* Joint effects of serum triglyceride and LDL cholesterol and HDL cholesterol concentrations on coronary heart disease risk in the Helsinki Heart Study: implication for treatment. *Circulation* 1992; **85**: 37–45.

20. Scandinavian Simvastatin Survival Study Group. Randomized trial of cholesterol lowering in 4444 patients with coronary heart disease: the Scandinavian Simvastatin Survival Study (4S). *Lancet* 1994; **344**: 1383–9.

21. Pedersen TR, Kjekshus J, Berg K, *et al.* Cholesterol lowering and the use of healthcare resources. Results of the Scandinavian Simvastatin Survival Study. *Circulation* 1996; **93**: 1796–802.

22. Byington RP, Jukema JA, Salonen JT, *et al.* Reduction in cardiovascular events during pravastatin therapy. Pooled analysis of clinical events of the Pravastatin Atherosclerosis Intervention Program. *Circulation* 1995; **92**: 2419–25.

23. Shepherd J, Cobbe SM, Ford I, Isles CG, Lorimer AR, MacFarlane PW, McKillop JH, Packard CJ. Prevention of coronary heart disease with pravastatin in men with hypercholesterolemia: West of Scotland Coronary Prevention Study group. *N Engl J Med* 1995; **333**: 1301–7.

24. Sacks FM, Pfeffer MA, Moye LA, *et al.* The effect of pravastatin on coronary events after myocardial infarction in patients with average cholesterol levels. Cholesterol and Recurrent Events Trial investigators. *N Engl J Med* 1996; **335**: 1001–9.

25. Haskell WL, Alderman EL, Fair JM, *et al.* Effects of intensive multiple risk factor reduction on coronary atherosclerosis and clinical cardiac events in men and women with coronary artery disease: the Stanford Coronary Risk Intervention Project (SCRIP). *Circulation* 1994; **89**: 975–90.

26. Blankenhorn DH, Nessim SA, Johnson RL, Sanmarcio ME, Azen SP, Cashin-Hemphill L. Beneficial effects of combined colestipol-niacin therapy on coronary atherosclerosis and coronary venous bypass grafts. *JAMA* 1987; **257**: 3233–40.

27. Blankenhorn DH, Azen SP, Kramsch DM, *et al.* Coronary angiographic changes with lovastatin therapy. The monitored atherosclerosis regression study (MARS). *Ann Intern Med* 1993; **119**: 969–76.

28. Brensike JF, Levy RI, Kelsey SF, *et al.* Effects of therapy with cholestyramine on progression of coronary atherosclerosis: results of the NHLBI Type II Coronary Intervention Study. *Circulation* 1984; **69**: 313–24.

29. Brown BG, Zhao XQ, Sacco DE, Albers JJ. Lipid lowering and plaque regression: new insights into prevention of plaque disruption and clinical events in coronary disease. *Circulation* 1993; **87**: 1781–91.

30. Brown BG, Albers JJ, Fisher LD, *et al.* Regression of coronary artery disease as a result of intensive lipid-lowering therapy in men with high levels of apolipoprotein B. *N Engl J Med* 1990; **323**: 1289–98.

31. Buchwald H, Varco RL, Matts JP, Long JM, Fitch LL, Campbell GS. Effect of partial ileal bypass surgery on mortality and morbidity from coronary heart disease in patients with

hypercholesterolemia: report of the Program on Surgical Control of the Hyperlipidemias (POSCH). *N Engl J Med* 1990; **323**: 946–55.

32. Fuster V, Badimon L, Badimon JJ, Chesbro JH. The pathogenesis of coronary artery disease and the acute coronary syndrome. *N Engl J Med* 1992; **326**: 242–56, 310–18.

33. Kane JP, Malloy MJ, Ports TA, Phillips NR, Diehl JC, Havel RJ. Regression of coronary atherosclerosis during treatment of familial hypercholesterolemia with combined drug regimens. *JAMA* 1990; **264**: 3007–12.

34. Watts GF, Lewis B, Brunt JNH, *et al*. Effects on coronary artery disease of lipid lowering diet: a diet plus cholestyramine in the St. Thomas Atherosclerosis Regression Study (STARS). *Lancet* 1992; **339**: 563–9.

35. Schuler G, Hambrecht R, Schlierf G, *et al*. Regular exercise and low fat diet: effects on progression of coronary artery disease. *Circulation* 1992; **86**: 1–11.

36. NIH Consensus Conference. Lowering blood cholesterol to prevent heart disease. *JAMA* 1985; **253**: 2080–6.

37. NIH Consensus Conference. Triglyceride, HDL cholesterol and coronary heart disease. *JAMA* 1993; 269: 505–10.

38. Gordon DJ, Knoke J, Probstfeld JL, Superko R, Tyroler HA. High density lipoprotein cholesterol and coronary heart disease in hypercholesterolemic men: the Lipid Research Clinics Coronary Primary Prevention Trial. *Circulation* 1986; **74**: 1217–25.

39. Gordon DJ, Rifkind BM. High-density lipoprotein: the clinical implications of recent studies. *N Engl J Med* 1989; **321**: 1311–16.

40. Rubins HB, Robins SJ, Collins D, Fye CL, Anderson JW, Elam MB, Faas FH, Linares E, Schaefer EJ, Schectman G, Wilt TJ, Wittes J, for the Veterans Affairs High-Density Lipoprotein Cholesterol Intervention Trial Study Group. Gemfibrozil for the secondary prevention of coronary heart disease in men with low levels of high-density lipoprotein cholesterol. *N Engl J Med* 1999; **341**: 410–18.

41. Robins SJ, Collins D, Wittes JT, Papademetriou V, Deedwania PC, Schaefer EJ, McNamara JR, Kashyap ML, Hershman JM, Wexler LF, Rubins HB; VA-HIT Study Group. Veterans Affairs High-Density Lipoprotein Intervention Trial. Relation of gemfibrozil treatment and lipid levels with major coronary events: VA-HIT: a randomized controlled trial. *JAMA* 2001; **285**: 1585–91.

42. Hokanson JE, Austin MA. Plasma triglyceride level as a risk factor for cardiovascular disease independent of high-density lipoprotein cholesterol level: a meta-analysis of population-based prospective studies. *J Cardiovasc Risk* 1996; **3**: 213–19.

43. Anderson KM, Wilson PWF, Odell PM, Kannel WB. An updated coronary risk profile. A statement for health professionals. AHA medical/scientific statement science advisory. *Circulation* 1991; **83**: 356–62.

44. Friedewald WT, Levy RI, Fredrickson DS. Estimation of the concentration of low density lipoproteins cholesterol without use of the preparative ultracentrifuge. *Clin Chem* 1972; **18**: 499–502.

45. Cooper GR, Myers GL, Smith SJ, Schlant RC. Blood lipid measurements. Variations and practical utility. *JAMA* 1992; **267**: 1652–60.

46. Tan MH, Wilmshurst EG, Gleason RE, Soldner JS. Effect of posture on serum lipids. *N Engl J Med* 1973; **289**: 416–19.

47. Warnick GR, Leary ET, Ammirati EB, Allen MP. Cholesterol in fingerstick capillary specimens can be equivalent to conventional venous measurements. *Arch Pathol Lab Med* 1994; **118**: 1110–14.

48. Genest JJ, Corbett H, McNamara JR, Schaefer MM, Salem DN, Schaefer EJ. Effect of hospitalization on high-density lipoprotein cholesterol in patients undergoing elective coronary angiography. *Am J Cardiol* 1988; **61**: 998–1000.

49. Genest JJ, McNamara JR, Ordovas JM, Martin-Munley S, Jenner JL, Millar J, Salem DN, Schaefer EJ. Effect of elective hospitalization on plasma lipoprotein cholesterol and apolipoproteins A-I, B and Lp(a). *Am J Cardiol* 1990; **65**: 677–9.

50. Laboratory Standardization Panel. National Cholesterol Education Program. Current status of blood cholesterol measurement in clinical laboratories in the United States: a report from the laboratory standardization panel of the National Cholesterol Education Program. *Clin Chem* 1988; **34**: 193–201.

51. Bachorik PS, Ross JW, for the National Cholesterol Education Program Working Group on Lipoprotein Measurement. National Cholesterol Education Program recommendations for measurement of low-density lipoprotein cholesterol: executive summary. *Clin Chem* 1995; **41**: 1414–20.

52. Stein EA, Myers GL, for the National Cholesterol Education Program Working Group on Lipoprotein Measurement. National Cholesterol Education Program recommendations for triglyceride measurement: executive summary. *Clin Chem* 1995; **41**: 1421–6.

53. Warnick GR, Wood PD JW, for the National Cholesterol Education Program Working Group on Lipoprotein Measurement. National Cholesterol Education Program recommendations for measurement of high-density lipoprotein cholesterol: executive summary. *Clin Chem* 1995; **41**: 1427–33.

54. McNamara JR, Cohn JS, Wilson PWF, Schaefer EJ. Calculated values for low density lipoprotein cholesterol in the assessment of lipid abnormalities and coronary disease risk. *Clin Chem* 1990; **36**: 36–42.

55. McNamara JR, Cole TG, Contois JH, Ferguson CA, Ordovas JM, Schaefer EJ. Immunoseparation method for measuring low-density lipoprotein cholesterol directly from serum evaluated. *Clin Chem* 1995; **41**: 232–40.

56. Jialal I, Hirany SV, Devaraj S, Sherwood TA. Comparison of an immunoseparation method for direct measurement of LDL-cholesterol with beta quantification (ultracentrifugation). *Am J Clin Path* 1995; **104**: 76–81.

57. Pisani T, Gepsky CP, Leary ET, Warnick GR, Ollington JF. Accurate direct determination of low-density lipoprotein cholesterol using an immunoseparation reagent and enzymatic cholesterol assay. *Arch Pathol Lab Med* 1995; **119**: 1127–35.

58. Nauck M, Rifai N. Analytical performance and clinical efficacy of three routine procedures for LDL cholesterol measurement compared with the ultracentrifugation dextran sulfate-Mg(2+) method. *Clin Chim Acta* 2000; **294**: 77–92.

59. Warnick GR, Nauck M, Rifai N. Evolution of methods for measurement of HDL-cholesterol: from ultracentrifugation to homogeneous assays. *Clin Chem* 2001; **47**: 1579–96.

60. Avogaro P, Bittolo Bon G, Cazzolato G, Quinci GB. Are apolipoproteins better discriminators than lipids for atherosclerosis? *Lancet* 1979; **1**: 901–3.

61. Sniderman A, Shapiro S, Marpole D, Skinner B, Teng B, Kwiterovich PO, Jr. Association of coronary atherosclerosis with hyperapobetalipoproteinemia (increased protein but normal cholesterol levels in human plasma low density lipoproteins). *Proc Natl Acad Sci USA* 1980; **77**: 604–8.

62. Whayne TF, Alaupovic P, Curry MD, Lee ET, Anderson PS, Snecter E. Plasma apolipoprotein B and VLDL-, LDL-, and HDL-cholesterol as risk factors in the development of coronary artery disease in male patients examined by angiography. *Atherosclerosis* 1981; **39**: 411–24.

63. Kwiterovich PO, Jr, Bachorik PS, Smith HH, *et al*. Hyperapobetalipoproteinaemia in two families with xanthomas and phytosterolaemia. *Lancet* 1981; **1**: 466–9.
64. Maciejko JJ, Holmes DR, Kottke BA, Zinsmeister AR, Dinh DM, Mao SJT. Apolipoprotein A-I as a marker of angiographically assessed coronary artery disease. *N Engl J Med* 1983; **309**: 385–9.
65. Genest JJ, Jr, McNamara JR, Ordovas JM, *et al*. Lipoprotein cholesterol, apolipoprotein A-I and B and lipoprotein(a) abnormalities in men with premature coronary artery disease. *J Am Coll Cardiol* 1992; **19**: 792–802.
66. Sigurdsson G, Baldursdottir A, Sigvalderson H, Agnarsson G, Thorgeirsson G, Sigfusson N. Predictive value of apolipoproteins in a prospective survey of coronary artery disease in men. *Am J Cardiol* 1992; **69**: 1251–4.
67. Ishikawa T, Fidge N, Thelle DS, Forde DH, Miller NE. The Tromso Heart Study: serum apolipoprotein A-I concentration in relation to future coronary heart disease. *Eur J Clin Invest* 1978; **8**: 179–82.
68. Salonen JT, Salonen R, Penttila I, *et al*. Serum fatty acids, apolipoproteins, selenium and vitamin antioxidants and the risk of death from coronary artery disease. *Am J Cardiol* 1985; **56**: 226–31.
69. Stampfer MJ, Sacks FM, Salvini S, Willett WC, Hennekens CH. A prospective study of cholesterol, apolipoproteins, and the risk of myocardial infarction. *N Engl J Med* 1991; **325**: 373–81.
70. Coleman MP, Key TJ, Wang DY, *et al*. A prospective study of obesity, lipids, apolipoproteins, and ischemic heart disease in women. *Atherosclerosis* 1992; **92**: 177–85.
71. Wald NJ, Law M, Watt HC, Wu T, Bailey A, Johnson AM, Craig WY, Ledue TB, Haddow JE. Apolipoproteins and ischaemic heart disease: implications for screening. *Lancet* 1994; **343**: 75–9.
72. Lamarche B, Despres JP, Moorjani S, Cantin B, Dagenais GR, Lupien P-J. Prevalence of dyslipidemic phenotypes in ischemic heart disease (prospective results from the Quebec Cardiovascular Study). *Am J Cardiol* 1995; **75**: 1189–95.
73. Marcovina SM, Albers JJ, Henderson LO, Hannon WH. International Federation of Clinical Chemistry standardization project for measurements of apolipoproteins A-I and B. III. Comparability of apolipoprotein A-I values by use of international reference material. *Clin Chem* 1993; **39**: 773–81.
74. Marcovina SM, Albers JJ, Kennedy H, Mei JV, Henderson LO, Hannon WH. International Federation of Clinical Chemistry standardization project for measurements of apolipoproteins A-I and B. IV. Comparability of apolipoprotein B values by use of international reference material. *Clin Chem* 1994; **40**: 586–92.
75. Contois JH, McNamara JR, Lammi-Keefe CJ, Wilson PWF, Schaefer EJ. Reference intervals for plasma apolipoprotein A-I as determined with a commercially available immunoturbidometric assay. Results from the Framingham Offspring Study. *Clin Chem* 1996; **42**: 507–14.
76. Contois JH, McNamara JR, Lammi-Keefe CJ, Wilson PWF, Schaefer EJ. Reference intervals for plasma apolipoprotein B as determined with a commercially available immunoturbidometric assay. Results from the Framingham Offspring Study. *Clin Chem* 1996; **42**: 515–23.
77. Sharrett AR, Ballantyne CM, Coady SA, Heiss G, Sorlie PD, Catellier D, Patsch W. Atherosclerosis Risk in Communities Study Group. Coronary heart disease prediction from lipoprotein cholesterol levels, triglycerides, lipoprotein(a), apolipoproteins A-I and B, and

HDL density subfractions: The Atherosclerosis Risk in Communities (ARIC) Study. *Circulation* 2001; **104**: 1108–13.

78. von Eckardstein A, Schulte H, Cullen P, Assmann G. Lipoprotein(a) further increases the risk of coronary events in men with high global cardiovascular risk. *J Am Coll Cardiol* 2001; **37**: 434–9.

79. Genest J, Jr, Jenner JL, McNamara JR, Ordovas JM, Silberman SR, Wilson PWF, Schaefer EJ. Prevalence of lipoprotein (a) [Lp(a)] excess in coronary artery disease. *Am J Cardiol* 1991; **67**: 1039–45.

80. Schaefer EJ, Lamon-Fava S, Jenner JL, *et al.* Lipoprotein(a) levels and risk of coronary heart disease in men. The Lipid Research Clinics Coronary Primary Prevention Trial. *JAMA* 1994; **271**: 999–1003.

81. Schwartzman RA, Cox ID, Poloniecki J, Crook R, Seymour CA, Kaski JC. Elevated plasma lipoprotein(a) is associated with coronary artery disease in patients with chronic stable angina pectoris. *J Am Coll Cardiol* 1998; **31**: 1260–6.

82. Dahlen GH, Stenlund H. Lp(a) lipoprotein is a major risk factor for cardiovascular disease: pathogenic mechanisms and clinical significance. *Clin Genet* 1997; **52**: 272–80.

83. Seman LJ, DeLuca C, Jenner JL, Cupples LA, McNamara JR, Wilson PWF, Castelli WP, Ordovas JM, Schaefer EJ. Lipoprotein(a)-cholesterol and coronary heart disease in the Framingham Heart Study. *Clin Chem* 1999; **45**: 1039–46.

84. Berg K, Dahlen G, Christophersen B, Cook T, Kjekshus J, Pedersen T. Lp(a) lipoprotein level predicts survival and major coronary events in the Scandinavian Simvastatin Survival Study. *Clin Genet* 1997; **52**: 254–61.

85. Bostom AG, Gagnon DR, Cupples LA, Wilson PWF, Jenner JL, Ordovas JM, Schaefer EJ, Castelli WP. A prospective investigation of elevated lipoprotein(a) detected by electrophoresis and cardiovascular disease in women. The Framingham Heart Study. *Circulation* 1994; **90**: 1688–95.

86. Bostom AG, Cupples LA, Jenner JL, Ordovas JM, Seman LJ, Wilson PWF, Schaefer EJ, Castelli WP. Elevated plasma Lp(a) and coronary heart disease in men aged 55 years and younger. A prospective study. *JAMA* 1996; **276**: 544–8.

87. Murai A, Miyahara T, Fujimoto N, Matsudo M, Kameyama M. Lp(a) lipoprotein as a risk factor for coronary heart disease and cerebral infarction. *Atherosclerosis* 1986; **59**: 199–204.

88. Sandkamp M, Funke H, Schulte H, Kohler E, Assmann G. Lipoprotein (a) is an independent risk factor for myocardial infarction at a young age. *Clin Chem* 1990; **36**: 20–3.

89. Rosengren A, Wihelmsen L, Eriksson E, Risberg B, Wedel H. Lipoprotein (a) and coronary heart disease: a prospective case-control study in the general population sample of middle aged men. *Br Med J* 1990; **301**: 1248–51.

90. Cremer P, Nagel D, Labrot B, Mann H, Muche R, Elster H, Seidel D. Lipoprotein Lp(a) as predictor of myocardial infarction in comparison to fibrinogen, LDL cholesterol and other risk factors: results from the prospective Gottingen Risk Incidence and Prevalence Study (GRIPS). *Eur J Clin Invest* 1994; **24**: 444–53.

91. Cantin B, Moorjani S, Dagenais GR, Lupien PJ. Lipoprotein(a) distribution in a French Canadian population and its relation to intermittent claudication (the Quebec Cardiovascular Study). *Am J Cardiol* 1995; **75**: 1224–8.

92. Assman G, Schulte H, von Eckardstein A. Hypertriglyceridemia and elevated lipoprotein(a) are risk factors for major coronary events in middle aged men. *Am J Cardiol* 1996; **77**: 1179–84.

93. Alfthan G, Pekkanen J, Juuhiainen M, Pitkaniemi J, Karvonen M, Tuomilehto J, Salonen JT, Ehnholm C. Relation of serum homocysteine and lipoprotein(a) concentrations to atherosclerotic disease in a prospective Finnish population based study. *Atherosclerosis* 1994; **106**: 9–19.

94. Ridker PM, Hennekens CH, Stampfer MJ. A prospective study of lipoprotein(a) and the risk of myocardial infarction. *JAMA* 1993; **270**: 2195–9.

95. Jauhiainen M, Koskinen P, Ehnholm C, *et al.* Lipoprotein (a) and coronary heart disease risk: a nested case-control study of the Helsinki Heart Study participants. *Atherosclerosis* 1991; **89**: 59–67.

96. Berg K. A new serum type system in man: the Lp system. *Acta Pathol Microbiol Scand* 1963; **59**: 369–82.

97. Utermann G. The mysteries of lipoprotein(a). *Science* 1989; **246**: 904–10.

98. Lackner C, Boerwinkle E, Leffert CC, Rahmig T, Hobbs HH. Molecular basis of apolipoprotein(a) isoform heterogeneity as revealed by pulsed-field gel electrophoresis. *J Clin Invest* 1991; **87**: 2153–61.

99. Boerwinkle E, Leffert CC, Lin J, Lackner C, Chiesa G, Hobbs HH. Apolipoprotein(a) gene accounts for greater than 90 percent of the variation in plasma lipoprotein(a) concentrations. *J Clin Invest* 1992; **90**: 52–60.

100. Marcovina SM, Koschinsky ML. Lipoprotein (a): Structure, measurement, and clinical significance. In: Rifai N, Warnick GR, eds. *Handbook of Lipoprotein Testing*. Washington, DC: AACC Press, 1997; 283–313.

101. McLean JW, Tomlinson JE, Kuang WJ, *et al.* cDNA sequence of human apolipoprotein(a) is homologous to plasminogen. *Nature* 1987; **330**: 132–7.

102. Hajjar KA, Gavish D, Breslow JL, Nachman RL. Lipoprotein(a) modulation of endothelial cell surface fibrinolysis and its potential role in atherosclerosis. *Nature* 1989; **339**: 303–5.

103. Loscalzo J, Weinfield M, Fless GM, Scanu AM. Lipoprotein(a), fibrin binding, and plasminogen activation. *Arteriosclerosis* 1990; **10**: 240–5.

104. Miles LA, Fless GM, Levin EG, Scanu AM, Plow EF. A potential basis for the thrombotic risks associated with lipoprotein(a). *Nature* 1989; **339**: 301–3.

105. Albers JJ, Adolphson JL, Hazzard WR. Radioimmunoassay of human plasma Lp(a) lipoprotein. *J Lipid Res* 1977; **18**: 331–8.

106. Seman LJ, Jenner JL, McNamara JR, Schaefer EJ. Quantitation of plasma lipoprotein (a) by cholesterol assay of lectin-bound lipoprotein (a). *Clin Chem* 1994; **40**: 400–3.

107. Jenner JL, Ordovas JM, Lamon-Fava S, Schaefer MM, Wilson PWF, Castelli WP, Schaefer EJ. Effects of age, sex, and menopausal status on plasma lipoprotein (a) levels. The Framingham Offspring Study. *Circulation* 1993; **87**: 1135–41.

108. Marcovina SM, Albers JJ, Jacobs DR, Jr, Perkins LL, Lewis CE, Howard BV, Savage P. Lipoprotein(a) concentrations and apolipoprotein(a) phenotypes in Caucasians and African Americans. The CARDIA Study. *Arterioscler Thromb* 1993; **13**: 1037–45.

109. Moliterno DJ, Jokinen EV, Miserez AR, Lange RA, Willard JE, Boerwinkle E, Hillis LD, Hobbs HH. No association between plasma lipoprotein(a) concentrations and the presence or absence of coronary atherosclerosis in African-Americans. *Arterioscler Thromb Vasc Biol* 1995; **15**: 850–5.

110. Schreiner PJ, Heiss G, Tyroler HA, Morrisett JD, Davis CE, Smith R. Race and gender differences in the association of Lp(a) with carotid artery wall thickness. The Atherosclerosis Risk in Communities (ARIC) Study. *Arterioscler Thromb Vasc Biol* 1996; **16**: 471–8.

111. Weiss SR, Bachorik PS, Becker LC, Moy TF, Becker DM. Lipoprotein(a) and coronary heart disease factors in a racially mixed population: the Johns Hopkins Sibling Study. *Ethn Dis* 1998; **8**: 60–72.

112. Seman LJ, McNamara JR, Schaefer EJ. Lipoprotein(a), homocysteine and remnant-like particles: emerging risk factors. *Curr Opin Cardiol* 1999; **14**: 186–91.

113. Canner PL, Berge KG, Wenger NK, Stamler J, Friedman L, Prineas RJ, Friedewald W. Fifteen-year mortality in Coronary Drug Project patients: long-term benefit with niacin. *J Am Coll Cardiol* 1986; **8**: 1245–55.

114. Carlson LA, Hamsten A, Asplund A. Pronounced lowering of serum lipoprotein Lp(a) in hyperlipidemic subjects treated with nicotinic acid. *J Intern Med* 1989; **226**: 271–6.

115. Cambien F, Jacqueson A, Richard JL, Warnet JM, Ducimetiere P, Claude JR. Is the level of serum triglyceride a significant predictor of coronary death in 'normocholesterolemic' subjects? The Paris Prospective Study. *Am J Epidemiol* 1986; **124**: 624–32.

116. Criqui MH, Heiss G, Cohn R, *et al*. Plasma triglyceride level and mortality from coronary heart disease. *N Engl J Med* 1993; **328**: 1220–5.

117. Hokanson JE, Austin MA. Plasma triglyceride level as a risk factor for cardiovascular disease independent of high-density lipoprotein cholesterol level: a meta-analysis of population-based prospective studies. *J Cardiovasc Risk* 1996; **3**: 213–19.

118. Miller M, Seidler A, Moalemi A, Pearson TA. Normal triglyceride levels and coronary artery disease events: the Baltimore Coronary Observational Long-Term Study. *J Am Coll Cardiol* 1998; **31**: 1252–7.

119. Doi H, Kugiyama K, Ohgushi M, *et al*. Remnants of chylomicron and very low density lipoprotein impair endothelium-dependent vasorelaxation. *Atherosclerosis* 1998; **137**: 341–9.

120. Mamo JC, Proctor SD, Smith D. Retention of chylomicron remnants by arterial tissue; importance of an efficient clearance mechanism from plasma. *Atherosclerosis* 1998; **141** (Suppl. 1): S63–9.

121. Ooi TC, Ooi DS. The atherogenic significance of an elevated plasma triglyceride level. *Crit Rev Clin Lab Sci* 1998; **35**: 489–516.

122. Havel RJ. Triglyceride-rich lipoproteins. In: Rifai N, Warnick GR, Dominiczak MH (eds), *Handbook of Lipoprotein Testing*, 3rd edn. Washington, DC: AACC Press 1997; 451–64.

123. Zilversmit DB. Atherogenesis: a postprandial phenomenon. *Circulation* 1979; **60**: 473–85.

124. Rapp JH, Lespine A, Hamilton RL, *et al*. Triglyceride-rich lipoproteins isolated by selected-affinity anti-apolipoprotein B immunosorption from human atherosclerotic plaque. *Arterioscler Thromb* 1994; **14**: 1767–74.

125. Karpe F, Taskinen MR, Nieminen MS, Frick MH, Kesaniemi YA, Pasternack A, Hamsten A, Syvanne M. Remnant-like lipoprotein particle cholesterol concentration and progression of coronary and vein-graft atherosclerosis in response to gemfibrozil treatment. *Atherosclerosis* 2001; **157**: 181–7.

126. Cohn JS. Postprandial lipemia: emerging evidence for atherogenicity of remnant lipoproteins. *Can J Cardiol* 1998; **14** (Suppl. B): 18B–27B.

127. Karpe F, Boquist S, Tang R, Bond GM, de Faire U, Hamsten A. Remnant lipoproteins are related to intima-media thickness of the carotid artery independently of LDL cholesterol and plasma triglycerides. *J Lipid Res* 2001; **42**: 17–21.

128. Cohn JS, McNamara JR, Cohn SD, Ordovas JM, Schaefer EJ. Plasma apolipoprotein changes in the triglyceride-rich lipoprotein fraction of human subjects fed a fat-rich meal. *J Lipid Res* 1988; **29**: 925–36.

129. Cohn JS, Johnson EJ, Millar JS, *et al*. Contribution of apoB-48 and apoB-100 triglyceride-rich lipoproteins (TRL) to postprandial increases in the plasma concentration of TRL triglycerides and retinyl esters. *J Lipid Res* 1993; **34**: 2033–40.

130. Karpe F, Hellenius ML, Hamsten A. Differences in postprandial concentrations of very-low-density lipoprotein and chylomicron remnants between normotriglyceridemic and hypertriglyceridemic men with and without coronary heart disease. *Metabolism* 1999; **48**: 301–7.

131. Campos E, Nakajima K, Tanaka A, Havel RJ. Properties of an apolipoprotein E-enriched fraction of triglyceride-rich lipoproteins isolated from human blood plasma with a monoclonal antibody to apolipoprotein B-100. *J Lipid Res* 1992; **33**: 369–80.

132. Nakajima K, Saito T, Tamura A, *et al*. Cholesterol in remnant-like lipoproteins in human serum using monoclonal anti apo B-100 and anti apo A-I immunoaffinity mixed gels. *Clin Chim Acta* 1993; **223**: 53–71.

133. Nakajima K, Okazaki M, Tanaka A, *et al*. Separation and determination of remnant-like particles in human serum using monoclonal antibodies to apo B-100 and apo A-I. *J Clin Ligand Assay* 1996; **19**: 177–83.

134. McNamara JR, Shah PK, Nakajima K, Cupples LA, Wilson PWF, Ordovas JM, Schaefer EJ. Remnant lipoprotein cholesterol and triglyceride reference ranges from the Framingham Heart Study. *Clin Chem* 1998; **44**: 1224–32.

135. Leary ET, Wang T, Baker DJ, Cilla DD, Zhong J, Warnick GR, Nakajima K, Havel RJ. Evaluation of an immunoseparation method for quantitative measurement of remnant-like particle-cholesterol in serum and plasma. *Clin Chem* 1998; **44**: 2490–8.

136. McNamara JR, Shah PK, Nakajima K, Cupples LA, Wilson PWF, Ordovas JM, Schaefer EJ. The association of remnant-like particle (RLP) cholesterol is an independent cardiovascular disease risk factor in women: results from the Framingham Heart Study. *Atherosclerosis* 2001; **154**: 229–37.

137. Takeichi S, Nakajima Y, Osawa M, Yukawa N, Saito T, Seto Y, Nakano T, Adachi M, Jitsukata K, Horiuchi K, Wang T, Nakajima K. The possible role of remnant-like particles as a risk factor for sudden cardiac death. *Int J Legal Med* 1997; **110**: 213–19.

138. Takeichi S, Yukawa N, Nakajima Y, *et al*. Association of plasma triglyceride-rich lipoprotein remnants with coronary atherosclerosis in cases of sudden cardiac death. *Atherosclerosis* 1999; **142**: 309–15.

139. Schaefer EJ, Audelin MC, McNamara JR, Shah PK, Tayler T, Daly JA, Augustin JL, Seman LJ, Rubenstein JJ. Comparison of fasting and postprandial plasma lipoproteins in subjects with and without coronary heart disease. *Am J Cardiol* 2001; **88**: 1129–33.

140. Shimizu H, Mori M, Saito T. An increase of serum remnant-like particles in non-insulin-dependent diabetic patients with microalbuminuria. *Clin Chim Acta* 1993; **221**: 191–6.

141. Nakajima K, Saito T, Tamura A, Suzuki M, Nakano T, Adachi M, Tanaka A, Tada N, Nakamura H, Murase T. A new approach for the detection of Type III hyperlipoproteinemia by RLP-cholesterol assay. *J Atheroscler Thromb* 1994; **1**: 30–6.

142. Devaraj S, Vega G, Lange R, Grundy SM, Jialal I. Remnant-like particle cholesterol levels in patients with dysbetalipoproteinemia or coronary artery disease. *Am J Med* 1998; **104**: 445–50.

143. McNamara JR, Shah PK, Tayler TD, Daly J, Ordovas JM, Schaefer EJ. Statin therapy reduces concentrations of remnant-like particles (Abstract). *Atherosclerosis* 1997; **134**: 346.

144. Mudd SH, Finkelstein JD. Homocysteinuria: an enzymatic defect. *Science* 1964; **143**: 1443–5.

145. Wilcken DEL, Wilcken B. The pathogenesis of coronary artery disease: a possible role for methionine metabolism. *J Clin Invest* 1976; **57**: 1079–94.
146. Yap S, Boers GH, Wilcken B, Wilcken DE, Brenton DP, Lee PJ, Walter JH, Howard PM, Naughten ER. Vascular outcome in patients with homocysteinuria due to cystathionine beta-synthase deficiency treated chronically: a multicenter observational study. *Arterioscler Thromb Vasc Biol* 2001; **21**: 2080–5.
147. Schnyder G, Roffi M, Pin R, Flammer Y, Lange H, Eberli FR, Meier B, Turi ZG, Hess OM. Decreased rate of coronary restenosis after lowering of plasma homocysteine levels. *N Engl J Med* 2001; **345**: 1593–600.
148. Genest JJ, Jr, McNamara JR, Salem DN, Wilson PWF, Schaefer EJ, Malinow MR. Plasma homocyst(e)ine levels in men with premature coronary artery disease. *J Am Coll Cardiol* 1990; **16**: 1114–19.
149. Stampfer MJ, Mallinow MR, Willett WC, *et al.* A prospective study of plasma homocyst(e)ine and risk of myocardial infarction in US physicians. *JAMA* 1991; **268**: 877–81.
150. Boushey CJ, Beresford SA, Omenn GS, Motulsky AG. A quantitative assessment of plasma homocysteine as a risk factor for vascular disease. Probable benefits of increasing folic acid intakes. *JAMA* 1995; **274**: 1049–57.
151. Rimm EB, Willett WC, Hu FB, Sampson L, Colditz GA, Manson JE, Hennekens C, Stampfer MJ. Folate and vitamin B6 from diet and supplements in relation to risk of coronary heart disease among women. *JAMA* 1998; **279**: 359–64.
152. Hoogeveen EK, Kostense PJ, Beks PJ, *et al.* Hyperhomocysteinemia is associated with an increased risk of cardiovascular disease, especially in non-insulin-dependent diabetes mellitus: a population-based study. *Arterioscler Thromb Vasc Biol* 1998; **18**: 133–8.
153. Donner MG, Klein GK, Mathes PB, Schwandt P, Richter WO. Plasma total homocysteine levels in patients with early-onset coronary heart disease and a low cardiovascular risk profile. *Metabolism* 1998; **47**: 273–9.
154. Folsom AR, Nieto FJ, McGovern PG, *et al.* Prospective study of coronary heart disease incidence in relation to fasting total homocysteine, related genetic polymorphisms, and B vitamins: the Atherosclerosis Risk in Communities (ARIC) study. *Circulation* 1998; **98**: 204–10.
155. Taylor LM, Jr, Moneta GL, Sexton GJ, Schuff RA, Porter JM. Prospective blinded study of the relationship between plasma homocysteine and progression of symptomatic peripheral arterial disease. *J Vasc Surg* 1999; **29**: 8–19.
156. Selhub J, Miller JW. The pathogenesis of homocysteinemia: interruption of the coordinate regulation by S-adenosylmethionine of the remethylation and transsulfuration of homocysteine. *Am J Clin Nutr* 1992; **55**: 131–8.
157. Lentz SR. Homocysteine and vascular dysfunction. *Life Sci* 1997; **61**: 1205–15.
158. Tyagi SC, Smiley LM, Mujumar VS, Clonts B, Parker JL. Reduction-oxidation (Redox) and vascular tissue level of homocyst(e)ine in human coronary atherosclerotic lesions and role in extracellular matrix remodeling and vascular tone. *Mol Cell Biochem* 1998; **181**: 107–16.
159. Genest J, Jr. Hyperhomocyst(e)inemia – determining factors and treatment. *Can J Cardiol* 1999; **15** (Suppl. B): 35B–38B.
160. Jacques PF, Rosenberg IH, Rogers G, *et al.* Serum total homocysteine concentrations in adolescent and adult Americans: results from the third National Health and Nutrition Examination Survey. *Am J Clin Nutr* 1999; **69**: 482–9.

161. Osganian SK, Stampfer MJ, Spiegelman D, *et al.* Distribution of and factors associated with serum homocysteine levels in children. Child and Adolescent Trial for Cardiovascular Health. *JAMA* 1999; **281**: 1189–96.

162. Selhub J, Jacques PF, Wilson PW, Rush D, Rosenberg IH. Vitamin status and intake as primary determinants of homocysteinemia in an elderly population. *JAMA* 1993; **270**: 2693–8.

163. Stehouwer CD, Weijenberg MP, van den Berg M, Jakobs C, Feskens EJ, Kromhout D. Serum homocysteine and risk of coronary heart disease and cerebrovascular disease in elderly men: a 10-year follow-up. *Arterioscler Thromb Vasc Biol* 1998; **18**: 1895–901.

164. Tucker KL, Mahnken B, Wilson PWF, Jaques P, Selhub J. Folic acid fortification of the food supply. Potential benefits and risks for the elderly population. *JAMA* 1996; **276**: 1879–85.

165. Chico A, Perez A, Cordoba A, *et al.* Plasma homocysteine is related to albumin excretion rate in patients with diabetes mellitus: a new link between diabetic nephropathy and cardiovascular disease? *Diabetologia* 1998; **41**: 684–93.

166. Bostom AG, Shemin D, Lapane KL, *et al.* Folate status is the major determinant of fasting total plasma homocysteine levels in maintenance dialysis patients. *Atherosclerosis* 1996; **123**: 193–202.

167. Hong SY, Yang DH, Chang SK. The relationship between plasma homocysteine and amino acid concentrations in patients with end-stage renal disease. *J Ren Nutr* 1998; **8**: 34–9.

168. Malinow MR, Duell PB, Hess DL, *et al.* Reduction of plasma homocyst(e)ine levels by breakfast cereal fortified with folic acid in patients with coronary heart disease. *N Engl J Med* 1998; **338**: 1009–15.

169. Hornberger J. A cost-benefit analysis of a cardiovascular disease prevention trial, using folate supplementation as an example. *Am J Public Health* 1998; **88**: 61–7.

170. Shipchandler MT, Moore EG. Rapid, fully automated measurement of plasma homocyst(e)ine with the Abbott IMx analyzer. *Clin Chem* 1995; **41**: 991–4.

171. Frantzen F, Faaren AL, Alfheim I, Nordhei AK. Enzyme conversion immunoassay for determining total homocysteine in plasma or serum. *Clin Chem* 1998; **44**: 311–16.

172. Ubbink JB, Delport R, Riezler R, Vermaak WJ. Comparison of three different plasma homocysteine assays with gas chromatography-mass spectrometry. *Clin Chem* 1999; **45**: 670–5.

173. Jacques PF, Bostom AG, Williams RR, Ellison RC, Eckfeldt JH, Rosenberg IH, Selhub J, Rozen R. Relation between folate status, a common mutation in methylenetetrahydrofolate reductase, and plasma homocysteine concentrations. *Circulation* 1996; **93**: 7–9.

174. McNamara JR, H. Campos JM, Ordovas J, Peterson PWF, Wilson EJ. Effect of gender, age, and lipid status on low density lipoprotein subfraction distribution: results from the Framingham Offspring Study. *Arteriosclerosis* 1987; **7**: 483–90.

175. Campos H, Blijlevens E, McNamara JR, Ordovas JM, Posner BM, Wilson PWF, Castelli WP, Schaefer EJ. LDL particle size distribution: results from the Framingham Offspring Study. *Arterioscler Thromb* 1992; **12**: 1410–19.

176. McNamara JR, Jenner JL, Li Z, Wilson PWF, Schaefer EJ. Change in low density lipoprotein particle size is associated with change in plasma triglyceride concentration. *Arterioscler Thromb* 1992; **12**: 1284–90.

177. Lamon-Fava S, Jimenez D, Christian JC, Fabsitz RR, Reed T, Carmelli D, Castelli WP, Ordovas JM, Wilson PWF, Schaefer EJ. The NHLBI Twin Study: heritability of apolipoprotein A-I, B and low density lipoprotein subclasses and concordance for lipoprotein (a). *Atherosclerosis* 1991; **91**: 97–106.

178. Austin MA, Breslow JL, Hennekens CH, Buring JE, Willett WC, Krauss RM. Low density lipoprotein subclass patterns and risk of myocardial infarction. *JAMA* 1988; **260**: 1917–21.

179. Rainwater DL, Martin LJ, Comuzzie AG. Genetic control of coordinated changes in HDL and LDL size phenotypes. *Arterioscler Thromb Vasc Biol* 2001; **21**: 1829–33.

180. Campos H, Genest JJ, Blijlevens E, *et al.* Low density lipoprotein particle size and coronary artery disease. *Arterioscler Thromb* 1992; **12**: 187–95.

181. McNamara JR, Small DM, Li Z, Schaefer EJ. Differences in LDL subspecies involve alterations in lipid composition and conformational changes in apolipoprotein B[1]. *J Lipid Res* 1996; **37**: 1924–35.

182. Freedman DS, Otvos JD, Jeyarajah EJ, Barboriak JJ, Anderson AJ, Walker JA. Relation of lipoprotein subclasses as measured by proton nuclear magnetic resonance spectroscopy to coronary artery disease. *Arterioscler Thromb Vasc Biol* 1998; **18**: 1046–53.

183. Stampfer MJ, Krauss RM, Ma J, Blanche PJ, Holl LG, Sacks FM, Hennekens CH. A prospective study of triglyceride level, low density lipoprotein particle diameter, and risk of myocardial infarction. *JAMA* 1996; **276**: 882–8.

184. St-Pierre AC, Ruel IL, Cantin B, Dagenais GR, Bernard PM, Despres JP, Lamarche B. Comparison of various electrophoretic characteristics of LDL particles and their relationship to the risk of ischemic heart disease. *Circulation* 2001; **104**: 2295–9.

185. Ford ES, Giles WH. Serum C-reactive protein and fibrinogen concentrations and self-reported angina pectoris and myocardial infarction: findings from National Health and Nutrition Examination Survey III. *J Clin Epidemiol* 2000; **53**: 95–102.

186. Blackburn R, Giral P, Bruckert E, Andre JM, Gonbert S, Bernard M, Chapman MJ, Turpin G. Elevated C-reactive protein constitutes an independent predictor of advanced carotid plaques in dyslipidemic subjects. *Arterioscler Thromb Vasc Biol* 2001; **21**: 1962–8.

187. Ridker PM, Hennekens CH, Buring JE, Rifai N. C-reactive protein and other markers of inflammation in the prediction of cardiovascular disease in women. *N Engl J Med* 2000; **342**: 836–43.

188. Haverkate F, Thompson SG, Pyke SD, Gallimore JR, Pepys MB. Production of C-reactive protein and risk of coronary events in stable and unstable angina. European Concerted Action on Thrombosis and Disabilities Angina Pectoris Study Group. *Lancet* 1997; **349**: 462–6.

189. Heeschen C, Hamm CW, Bruemmer J, Simoons ML. Predictive value of C-reactive protein and troponin T in patients with unstable angina: a comparative analysis. CAPTURE Investigators. Chimeric c7E3 AntiPlatelet Therapy in Unstable angina REfractory to standard treatment trial. *J Am Coll Cardiol* 2000; **35**: 1535–42.

190. Ridker PM, Cushman M, Stampfer MJ, Tracy RP, Hennekens CH. Inflammation, aspirin, and the risk of cardiovascular disease in apparently healthy men. *N Engl J Med* 1997; **336**: 973–9.

191. Hak AE, Pols HA, Stehouwer CD, Meijer J, Kiliaan AJ, Hofman A, Breteler MM, Witteman JC. Markers of inflammation and cellular adhesion molecules in relation to insulin resistance in nondiabetic elderly: the Rotterdam study. *J Clin Endocrinol Metab* 2001; **86**: 4398–405.

192. Albert MA, Danielson E, Rifai N, Ridker PM; PRINCE Investigators. Effect of statin therapy on C-reactive protein levels: the pravastatin inflammation/CRP evaluation (PRINCE): a randomized trial and cohort study. *JAMA* 2001; **286**: 64–70.

193. Macy EM, Hayes TE, Tracy RP. Variability in the measurement of C-reactive protein in healthy subjects: implications for reference intervals and epidemiological applications. *Clin Chem* 1997; **43**: 52–8.

194. Rifai N, Tracy RP, Ridker PM. Clinical efficacy of an automated high-sensitivity C-reactive protein assay. *Clin Chem* 1999; **45**: 2136–41.
195. Wilkins J, Gallimore JR, Moore EG, Pepys MB. Rapid automated high sensitivity enzyme immunoassay of C-reactive protein. [Technical Brief]. *Clin Chem* 1998; **44**: 1358–61.

6

Who to treat?

SANJEEV PURI AND JEROME D COHEN

INTRODUCTION

It is well established that high levels of low-density lipoprotein (LDL)-cholesterol play the central role in the development of atherosclerotic disease, and major advances have been made during the past 20 years in understanding the pathogenesis of the disease. Physicians have aggressively pursued the application of new diagnostic and interventional techniques and new pharmacological approaches to minimize myocardial injury or the effects of ischemia, but this enthusiasm for the treatment of ischemia has not been paralleled by the application of proven measures aimed at prevention, both primary and secondary. In the United States, coronary heart disease (CHD) accounts for an estimated 500 000 deaths each year, and stroke for another 140 000 deaths; moreover, among survivors the vast majority will subsequently die from their disease.[1] Taken together, cardiovascular diseases kill Americans at the rate of one every 34 s. Further, first-event sudden death is responsible for approximately 30 percent of all coronary deaths.

Americans are leading the world in terms of cholesterol awareness, and the US population mean cholesterol level has shown a consistent decline over the past 25 years.[2] This decline in cholesterol levels, reflecting dietary changes, coupled with the impressive decrease in cigarette smoking has been estimated to have contributed substantially to the decrease in CHD mortality and morbidity observed over the past two decades.[3] However, the sobering statistics cited above underscore the rationale and need for effective prevention strategies for further reducing the morbidity and mortality associated with CHD.

In this chapter, we will review the guidelines for identifying and treating patients with high cholesterol and compare the NCEP guidelines to those of the ACP, Canadian Preventive Task Force, and the European Task Force.[4-7] We will also discuss guidelines for management of lipid disorders in special population groups, including patients with average cholesterol levels, elderly, women, diabetics, and minorities.

ASSESSMENT OF CHD RISK STATUS

The intensity of the treatment of an individual patient depends on the overall assessment of risk. The basic principle is that those at higher risk should be targeted for more aggressive treatment than those at lower risk. Since CHD is multifactorial in its origin, it is important when estimating the risk of CHD for an individual to take into consideration overall cardiovascular risk. At any given level of serum cholesterol, an individual with two or more risk factors is at higher risk than an individual without other risk factors present. Overall cardiovascular risk can be estimated by using tables, dedicated risk calculators, or computer programs. As an illustration of one approach, a simplified method of deriving an approximate CHD risk function derived from the Framingham data is commonly used.[8] This Coronary Risk Chart has been simplified in many ways to facilitate use; for example, total cholesterol rather than LDL-cholesterol (LDL-C) is used. The level of systolic blood pressure is tracked vertically, and the cholesterol level is tracked horizontally. Using the appropriate sections for age, sex, and smoking status, an approximate estimate for absolute 10-year risk of a CHD event can be determined. Subjects with diabetes, established CHD, or peripheral vascular disease are at higher risk and should be moved up one risk category.

In 1993, the National Cholesterol Education Program (NCEP) published revised guidelines for risk assessment and patient stratification. In 2001, another update was released (see Chapter 11); these are shown in Box 6.1. The major changes from the original guidelines include consideration of age and gender in risk assessment. Men, aged 45 years and older, and women over the age of 55 years or postmenopausal

---

Box 6.1 *NCEP – ATP III risk algorithm*

Major risk factors (exclusive of LDL cholesterol) that modify LDL goals:

- Cigarette smoking
- Hypertension (blood pressure ≥140/90 mmHg or on antihypertensive medication).
- Low HDL cholesterol (<40 mg/dL)[a]
- Family history of premature CHD (CHS in male first-degree relative <55 years; CHD in female first-degree relative <65 years)
- Age (men ≥45 years; women ≥55 years)

Diabetes is regarded as a coronary heart disease (CHD) risk equivalent. LDL indicates low–density lipoprotein; HDL, high–density lipoprotein.
[a]HDL cholesterol >60 mg/dl counts as a 'negative' risk factor; its presence removes 1 risk factor from the total count.

women of any age without estrogen replacement therapy are identified as being at higher risk. Patients with non-coronary atherosclerotic vascular disease [transient ischemic attack (TIA), thrombotic stroke, intermittent claudication] have been targeted along with coronary patients for secondary prevention. The guidelines define three levels of CHD risk:

1. Those at highest risk for future CHD events because of known CHD or other atherosclerotic disease (secondary prevention).
2. Patients without evident CHD who have two or more risk factors.
3. Patients with less than two additional risk factors.

The last group includes young adult men (under 35 years of age) and pre-menopausal women. The guidelines also define three categories of risk based on the serum total cholesterol. Serum cholesterol levels less than 200 mg/dL are 'desirable'; those between 200 and 239 mg/dL are designated 'borderline high'; and levels greater than 240 mg/dL are defined as 'high.' About 40 percent of the adult American population has desirable levels; 40 percent has borderline high levels; and the remaining 20 percent has high concentrations.[9] Importantly, based on the randomized clinical trial data, the LDL-C level is used as the guide for therapy and is the primary target for intervention. Therefore, the classification is further refined based on the LDL-C levels and is shown in Table 6.1. Because of the inverse relationship between high-density lipoprotein-cholesterol (HDL-C) concentration

Table 6.1 *LDL cholesterol goals and cutpoints for Therapeutic Lifestyle Changes (TLC) and drug therapy in different risk categories*[a]

Risk category	LDL goal	LDL level at which to initiate therapeutic lifestyle changes	LDL level at which to consider drug therapy
CHD or CHD risk equivalents (10-year risk >20%)	<100	≥100	≥130 (100–129: drug optional)[b]
2+Risk factors (10-year risk ≤20%)	<130	≥130	10-year risk 10%–20%: ≥130 10-year risk <10%: ≥160
0–1 Risk factor[c]	<160	≥160	≥190 (160–189: LDL-lowering drug optional)

Values are mg/dL.
[a]LDL indicates low-density lipoprotein; coronary heart disease.
[b]Some authorities recommend use of LDL-lowering drugs in this category if an LDL cholesterol level of <100 mg/dL cannot be achieved by therapeutic lifestyle changes. Others prefer use of drugs that primarily modify triglycerides and HDL, e.g. nicotinic acid or fibrate. Clinical judgment also may call for deferring drug therapy in this subcategory.
[c]Almost all people with 0–1 risk factor have a 10-year risk <10%; thus, 10-year risk assessment in people with 0–1 risk factor is not necessary.

and CHD risk, a low HDL-C (<35 mg/dL) is regarded as a positive risk factor, and a high level of HDL-C (>60 mg/dL) is considered a negative risk factor.

SCREENING

Issues regarding the screening of the general population for hypercholesterolemia focus on two basic questions: (i) whom to screen?; and (ii) how to screen? There is little – if any – debate regarding patients with known CHD or other forms of atherosclerotic vascular disease. On the other hand, there has been considerable debate over the best strategy to identify hypercholesterolemia among asymptomatic people. The NCEP recommends that all adults aged 20 years or more have serum total cholesterol measured at least once every 5 years; HDL-C should be measured at the same time. This is a more aggressive strategy than the ACP guidelines in which screening is recommended only for men aged over 35 years and women aged over 45 years. The Canadian task force took gender into consideration and recommended screening of all men aged between 30 and 59 years. The European guidelines rely on risk of CHD, and do not provide age-specific guidelines. Screening at a younger age is recommended for earlier identification of a relatively high-risk population and helps to focus attention on high levels of blood cholesterol as a major CHD risk factor and the need and desirability for more aggressive subsequent lifestyle modification. These recommendations are prudent in view of the data from the West of Scotland Coronary Prevention Study (WOSCOPS) trial.[10]

Not only are there differences in the guidelines regarding screening in the younger population, but there is also controversy over screening of the elderly population. The aggressive approach recommended by the NCEP is based on the rationale that the prevalence and incidence of atherosclerosis is much more common in older age groups, and CVD is, by far, the most common cause of death among older Americans. However, some experts challenge the wisdom of aggressive screening of the elderly citing insufficient evidence to justify the cost and socioeconomic implications of this approach.[11] With the established safety of hexamethylglutaryl-coenzyme A (HMG-CoA) reductase inhibitors and because of the significant risk of CHD in the elderly, appropriate screening should be implemented in this population. Older patients should not be denied the proven benefits of lipid-lowering which include not only CHD, but also stroke reduction.

The second question is *how* to screen. According to NCEP guidelines, initial screening begins with the measurement of total cholesterol and HDL-C levels, and these can be measured in a non-fasting state as neither the total nor the HDL-C levels change significantly after meals. It is preferable to collect serum because the cholesterol values cited in the various guidelines are for serum; plasma levels are generally lower by about 3 percent. Lipoprotein analysis usually provides measured results for total cholesterol, HDL-C and triglycerides, and LDL-C is calculated using the Friedwald formula when triglycerides (TG) are less than 400 mg/dL.[12] If a fasting lipoprotein profile can be obtained initially, this can save the patient the time and expense of returning for follow-up. The cost differential of measuring HDL-C and triglycerides is small compared to the value of the information acquired.

A high level of LDL-C is the major atherogenic factor, and it can be measured directly in the non-fasting state using an immunoseparation assay. This direct assay is of great value when triglyceride levels exceed 400 mg/dL – levels at which LDL-C is not estimated because the formula is not reliable. The direct method of LDL-C measurement is accurate even in the presence of hypertriglyceridemia, and it is highly recommended for laboratories to perform this test reflexively when TG levels exceed 400 mg/dL or if the patient is non-fasting. Recent evidence suggests that direct LDL-C measurement may be superior when triglycerides exceed 250 mg/dL because the calculated LDL-C level at TG levels of 250–400 mg/dL results in significant patient misclassification.[13]

SCREENING FOR PRIMARY PREVENTION

Primary prevention refers to preventing clinical manifestations among people who do not yet have clinical evidence of disease. Two basic approaches can be taken for primary prevention:

• the high-risk individual strategy for the identification of high-risk individuals as advocated by the NCEP; and
• a public health approach, which is a population-based strategy aimed at modifying lifestyle habits of the general population to reduce overall CHD risk.

The high-risk individual strategy is based on two observations. First, the upper portion of the population distribution accounts for a disproportionate share of the disease; and second, the relationship between blood cholesterol levels and coronary disease is not linear but exponential (Figure 6.1).[14,15] Treatment focusing only on the high-risk group will lead to considerable benefit in CHD reduction, but benefits will be limited to this high-risk group. On the other hand, using population-based strategies, a small shift in the mean cholesterol will be spread across the entire population, leading to a potentially large overall CHD reduction. These two approaches are not mutually exclusive but are complementary. Hence, both should be pursued with vigor to derive the most effective CHD prevention.

A large database indicates that, on average, for every 1 percent change in cholesterol levels the risk of CHD changes by 2 percent.[16,17] The epidemiological literature suggests that this may be an underestimate of this relationship, and the change in CHD risk may be 3 percent for every 1 percent reduction in cholesterol.[18] The controversy which arose from the results of early primary prevention trials stemmed not only from the question of efficacy but also from concerns about safety and the impact on overall mortality. Gould and colleagues suggested that specific adverse effects which offset much of the benefit of the reduction of coronary risk in the early primary prevention trials were confined to treatment with hormones and fibrates, and no trial had shown a decrease in total mortality.[19] In the West of Scotland Coronary Prevention Study, a 26 percent reduction in the LDL-C level by pravastatin treatment led to a 31 percent reduction in non-fatal myocardial infarction (MI), 32 percent reduction in death from all cardiovascular causes, and a 22 percent reduction in risk of death from any cause.[11] With these landmark trials

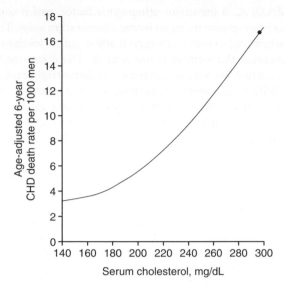

Figure 6.1 *Relationship of serum cholesterol to coronary heart disease death in 361 662 men aged 35–57 years during an average follow-up of 6 years in MRFIT screenees. Each point represents a median value for 5% of the population. Key points are as follows: (i) risk increases steadily, particularly above levels of 200 mg/dL; and (ii) magnitude of increased risk is large, four-fold in the top 10% when compared with the bottom 10%. Reproduced from Reference 15, with permission.*

and the safety data from the Scandinavian Simvastatin Survival Study (4S), Cholesterol And Recurrent Events (CARE) and LIPID secondary prevention trials, concerns about the overall efficacy and safety of cholesterol-lowering, using statins, have been reduced.

As per the NCEP guidelines shown in Table 6.1, the target goal for patients without CHD or other forms of atherosclerotic disease is an LDL-C level <160 mg/dL when there are fewer than two risk factors present, and <130 mg/dL in the presence of two or more other risk factors.[4] Lifestyle changes focusing on diet and augmented by increased physical activity are the cornerstone of therapy and should be initiated in every patient. Lipid-lowering drug therapy should be considered after a trial of diet therapy. In accordance with the NCEP guidelines, LDL-C levels >190 mg/dL in the absence of two other risk factors, or LDL-C levels >160 mg/dL in the presence of two or more risk factors, should be targeted for pharmacotherapy. A concern has been expressed about the wisdom of the NCEP guidelines regarding drug treatment in younger adult men aged less than 35 years and in premenopausal females with no risk factors but who have LDL-C values in the 190–220 mg/dL range. The Air Force/Texas Coronary Atherosclerosis Prevention Study (AFCAPS/TexCAPS) is a landmark primary prevention trial. It included 6605 healthy men and women with average total cholesterol (mean TC: 221 mg/dL; LDL-C: 150 mg/dL) that was considerably less than that in the West of Scotland trial, and below average HDL-C (mean for men 36 mg/dL; for women 40 mg/dL). After 5.2 years of treatment with lovastatin, the incidence of major acute coronary heart disease events (fatal or non-fatal MI, unstable angina or sudden cardiac death) was reduced by 37 percent (p <0.001), in absolute terms from 10.9 percent to 6.8 percent.[11A] A prudent approach is to consider drug therapy in younger patients with genetic dyslipidemia and a strong family history of premature coronary artery disease (CAD) or diabetes mellitus. In the Canadian guidelines the important difference from the NCEP guidelines is that recommendations for primary prevention are only made for asymptomatic men aged between 30 and 59 years.[6] The European guidelines place emphasis on the estimation of absolute CHD risk as a determinant for lipid management, and the initial screening is based on total cholesterol number. When the absolute CHD risk is >20 percent based on the coronary risk chart, fasting TC, LDL-C, HDL-C and triglyercides are measured and an initial lifestyle modification for 3 months is recommended with repeat lipid measurements. Drug therapy is recommended to achieve TC <190 mg/dL and LDL-C <115 mg/dL if lifestyle advice fails. The WOSCOPS and AFCAPS/TexCAPS provided strong evidence for the benefits of primary prevention through lipid-regulating treatment, as well as the safety of statin therapy. The AFCAPS/TexCAPS data extend the benefits to a large segment of population at risk for a first CHD event. In contrast to WOSCOPS, only 17 percent of AFCAPS/TexCAPS participants would have met NCEP criteria for drug therapy. It is likely that future guidelines will favor more aggressive reduction of LDL-C for primary prevention. The cost-effectiveness of such an approach has been the subject of much debate, but undoubtedly will improve in the future as the cost of lipid-lowering drugs falls.

SCREENING FOR SECONDARY PREVENTION

More than 1 million cases of MI occur each year, and the vast majority of patients survive the acute event. Subsequent mortality rates are greatest during the first year, and thereafter the annual recurrence rate – death or non-fatal MI – is around 5 percent for men and 7 percent for women.[20] After a first infarction, the risk of subsequent infarction is increased three- to six-fold over age- or gender-matched individuals who have not had a prior infarct. The risk of any cardiovascular event occurring within 5 years of a MI is as high as 80 percent.[21] The presence of angina pectoris doubles the relative risk of subsequent CHD mortality, and the risk of non-coronary events is also increased. Patients with symptomatic CHD have an ischemic stroke rate of 1–2 percent per year – a rate which falls between that seen in age- or gender-matched general population and those with a previous history of TIA or stroke.[22] Similarly, patients with other forms of atherosclerotic disease – either cerebrovascular or peripheral vascular disease – have a four- to six-fold higher risk of CHD as compared with the general population. In this high-risk group of CHD patients, landmark clinical trials have shown significant reduction in event rates. The 4S study was the first to show a significant (30%) reduction in total mortality, solely due to a reduction in fatal cardiac events.[23] The baseline total cholesterol was 260 mg/dL and LDL-C was 188 mg/dL, and these were reduced in the active treatment group by 25 percent and 35 percent, respectively. The decrease in total mortality is noteworthy because of the prior concern about higher non-cardiovascular mortality rates based on non-significant trends observed in previous studies.

The NCEP guidelines for secondary prevention (see Table 6.1) indicate an LDL-C level of 100 mg/dL or lower as the goal of therapy. Drug therapy is indicated in patients with established CHD or other atherosclerotic disease if the LDL-C level is 130 mg/dL (3.4 mmol/L) or greater after diet therapy. If the level is between 100 and 129 mg/dL, clinical judgment should be used to weigh potential benefits versus side effects and cost. However, given the consistent findings for the benefits and relative safety of lipid-lowering therapy – and specifically for the statins – it appears most prudent to pursue aggressively any lipid lowering by pharmacotherapy in this group of patients. Furthermore, it may be in the patients' best interest not to wait for a 3- or 6-month trial period of dietary intervention. This is based on the observation that the vast majority of patients will not achieve the recommended LDL-C goal by diet therapy alone, and the window of opportunity for initiation of drugs with maximum patient compliance may not extend to 3 or 6 months. Likewise, if LDL-C is between 100 and 129 mg/dL on a single drug, increasing the dose or adding a second agent to reduce the level to below 100 mg/dL requires careful consideration. The recent publication of the post-coronary artery bypass grafting (CABG) trial results compared a regimen of moderate LDL-C reduction (130–140 mg/dL) to a more aggressive regimen (60–85 mg/dL) in patients who had undergone CABG previously.[24] Patients with aggressive lowering of LDL-C had a 31 percent reduction in the likelihood of progression of graft atherosclerosis and occlusion as compared with the moderate treatment group. The trial lacked statistical power to examine the effect on clinical events, but the trend was favorable – a 29 percent reduction in the rate of revascularization in the aggressive treatment group.

PATIENTS WITH CAD AND AVERAGE CHOLESTEROL

A large proportion of patients with CAD have cholesterol levels which are in the average range.[2] The CARE trial examined the effectiveness of cholesterol-lowering therapy with pravastatin in a post-MI population with a mean cholesterol level of 209 mg/dL and a mean LDL-C of 139 mg/dL.[25] These patients represent approximately 75 percent of post-MI patients, with total cholesterols ranging from 180 to 239 mg/dL and LDL-Cs from 115 to 174 mg/dL. On-treatment reductions were 20 percent and 28 percent, respectively, and resulted in a 24 percent reduction in recurrent events (non-fatal MI or CHD death).

Despite the success of these recent clinical trials in decreasing the morbidity and mortality in CAD with reduction of LDL-C, there remains a substantial population which has manifest CAD with LDL-C levels in the average or lower-than average range. Although there were significantly fewer clinical events in the active treatment groups, there was still a considerable number of patients who, despite LDL-C reduction, had progression of CAD or experienced a clinical event.[26] Patients who have plasma total cholesterol and LDL-C in the average or 'normal' range may have other lipid abnormalities that may contribute to the atherosclerotic process. Among other factors, consideration should be given to the atherogenic lipid profile (ALP), lipoprotein(a) (Lp(a)), and homocysteinemia.[27,28]

Atherogenic lipoprotein profile

The ALP is characterized by a predominance of small, dense LDL-C particles (also called LDL-C subclass pattern B), low levels of HDL-C, high triglyceride levels, post-prandial hyperlipidemia, insulin resistance, and abdominal obesity.[26,27] The ALP is a heritable trait composed of these metabolic features which leads to an atherogenic milieu. The high CAD risk associated with ALP has been demonstrated in the Boston Area Health Project, the prospective Physicians Health Survey, and the Stanford Five City Project – all of which showed ALP to be associated with a three-fold increased risk of CAD independent of other risk factors including total cholesterol, HDL-C, apolipoprotein B, and body mass index.[29,30] The prospective Québec Cardiovascular Study also showed that high levels of small, dense LDL-C particles (pattern B) were associated with increased risk of subsequent development of CAD in men, independent of the plasma lipid concentrations.[31] A number of angiographic trials have demonstrated that the progression of atherosclerotic lesions, and subsequent clinical event rates, were significantly correlated with changes in intermediate density lipoprotein (IDL) and HDL-C. Elevated IDL and low levels of HDL-C are also characteristic of ALP. Additional prospective studies are needed to define the exact role of ALP in atherosclerosis and the effects of treatment, particularly among those patients who have relatively low levels of LDL-C. Problems with laboratory measurements also need to be solved since, until these issues are resolved, routine screening for LDL-C subclasses is not recommended.

Lipoprotein(a)

Lipoprotein(a) is an LDL-C-like particle which contains a unique apolipoprotein called apo(a). Apo(a) is similar in part to plasminogen and may interfere with plasminogen activation. Among the major lipoprotein classes, Lp(a) appears to have the highest gene linkage, with the apo(a) gene locus accounting for 90 percent of the variability in blood levels.[32] The distribution of Lp(a) is skewed to the left in most populations, and a value >30 mg/dL is considered to be elevated. Afro-Americans show a bell-shaped distribution curve with higher Lp(a) values overall. Numerous retrospective and prospective studies have implicated Lp(a) as a strong risk factor for the development of premature CAD, not only in patients with elevated LDL-C but also in those with average LDL-C levels.[28] Performing Lp(a) analysis with precision and good reproducibility is difficult, and analyses only should be carried out by experienced laboratories. The treatment of elevated Lp(a) is problematic; the only drugs shown to have some impact are nicotinic acid, estrogens, and bezafibrate. No prospective clinical trials have shown that lowering of high levels of Lp(a) reduces CAD incidence. At the present time, measurement of Lp(a) should be considered in screening patients with high risk of premature CHD, and patients with CHD but 'normal' lipid levels.

Box 6.2 *Lp(a) testing*

Measurement:
- Lp(a) can be measured by its total mass [Lp(a)] or by its cholesterol content [Lp (a)-C]
- Lp(a) assays are now available with FDA clearance (monoclonal antibody-based quantitative ELISA)

Who to test:
Primary prevention
- Family history of premature atherosclerosis not explained by other dyslipidemias
- Hypercholesterolemia, not responsive to cholesterol-lowering therapy (statins or bile acid sequestrants)

Secondary prevention
- Premature atherosclerosis˙
- Revascularization (CABG/PTCA) patients – restenosis
- Heart transplant recipients

Values:	*Mass*	*Cholesterol*
High-risk	>30 mg/dL	>10 mg/dL
Borderline high-risk	20–30 mg/dL	5–10 mg/dL
Desirable	<20 mg/dL	<5 mg/dL

Treatment:
- Take more aggressive action to reduce modifiable risk factors (i.e. smoking, hypertension)
- Niacin
- Estrogen therapy for postmenopausal women

˙Several leading lipid specialists now recommend testing anyone with atherosclerosis for Lp(a).

Homocysteine

Elevated levels of homocysteine are considered to be an independent risk factor for premature coronary, peripheral vascular, and cerebrovascular disease.[33,34] Two large prospective, observational studies – The Physicians Health Study and a Norwegian study – found higher baseline homocysteine levels among those patients who subsequently developed an MI than among those who did not.[35,36] Elevations in homocysteine can be caused both by genetic and nutritional factors. The exact mechanism of high levels of homocysteine in the development of atherosclerosis is unknown, but possibilities include adverse effects on the endothelium, platelets, and clotting factors. There may also be an interaction between high homocysteine levels and LDL-C. Although treatment is readily available with folic acid, no randomized clinical trials have studied the effects of the treatment of high homocysteine on cardiovascular morbidity and mortality. Until such data are available, routine screening for high levels of homocysteine is not indicated, but it may be useful in selected patients with normal lipoprotein fractions who have atherosclerotic disease and/or a strong family history.

Box 6.3 *Homocysteine testing*

Measurement:
- Generally determined using high-performance liquid chromatography
- New methods include chemiluminescence and colorimetric assays

Who to test:
Secondary prevention
- Patients with atherosclerosis – with few standard risk factors
- Revascularization (CABG/PTCA) patients – restenosis
- Heart transplant recipients

Values: High risk   >19 µmol/L
                Average   6–16 µmol/L
                Desirable   <6.3 µmol/L

Treatment:
- Vitamin supplementation, especially folic acid, vitamin B_6 and vitamin B_1

Elderly

Controversy persists regarding the screening for, and treatment of, hyperlipidemia in patients aged over 65 years, primarily because of the paucity of data. Most earlier lipid-lowering studies excluded the participation of older patients. Reviews of data obtained from prospective epidemiological studies have shown an association in one or both sexes between serum total cholesterol and CHD in persons aged over 65 years.[37] The relative risk of elevated cholesterol continues to predict coronary disease, although the strength of this relationship decreases with increasing age. This is due to the fact that, as the population ages, the proportion of deaths from CVD increases across the entire range of cholesterol levels. The relative risk of higher versus lower cholesterol levels (the ratio) is thereby decreased. Of greater importance for screening and treatment considerations is the absolute attributable risk, the excess disease due to high levels of cholesterol which increases with age.[38] The incidence and number of events associated with higher versus lower levels of cholesterol increases, and therefore the total number of people potentially benefiting from cholesterol lowering will be greater in the older population.[37]

The recent 4S study enrolled 52 percent of patients aged over 60 years. Analysis of the benefit seen in this older group indicated a 27 percent reduction in mortality (p <0.01) and a 29 percent reduction in risk for major coronary events (p <0.0001), similar to the results for the younger cohort.[23] In the CARE study, treatment with pravastatin in the older compared with the younger participants resulted in a greater absolute benefit with regard to major cardiovascular events.[25] The WOSCOP study included patients about half of whom were aged between 55 and 65 years. The risk of non-fatal MI or death was reduced by 27 percent (p <0.0089) in this older group compared with 40 percent (p <0.0024) in the younger patients, but this difference was not statistically significant.[11] The AFCAPS/TexCAPS cohort had 21 percent of participants aged over 65 years, and showed significant benefit from drug therapy. It is clear from these recent randomized clinical trials that chronological age in and of itself should not be a reason to withhold lipid-lowering therapy.

The NCEP guidelines urge caution regarding the use of lipid-lowering medications in the elderly.[4] Treatment decisions in the elderly need to be based on careful evaluation of the overall health and medical condition of the patient. This is more difficult in this age group as they often have co-morbid conditions. Aggressive lipid lowering may be ill-advised in an elderly person who has a significant competing illness, with limited life expectancy. On the other hand, most elderly patients are free-living and in relatively good health. In view of the excellent results of secondary prevention trials, aggressive lipid-lowering in elderly patients is recommended unless otherwise contra-indicated. For primary prevention, a more conservative approach to lipid lowering involving diet and exercise therapy, to the extent possible, should be followed. Lipid-lowering therapy should also be considered in an otherwise healthy elderly patient with multiple risk factors. An additional benefit of lipid lowering which is of great interest and concern to elderly patients, is the reduction in the incidence of stroke. In the CARE trial, stroke – a specified endpoint – was reduced by 31 percent.[25] Similar results have been observed in trials with niacin and simvastatin.

Women

Although not widely recognized, CAD is the most common cause of death in women. Indeed, after the age of 55 years, more deaths occur among women from CAD than from all cancers combined.[39] However, premenopausal women with hypercholesterolemia generally have a low absolute risk of CHD and, in the absence of atherosclerotic disease or multiple risk factors, a conservative approach involving diet and exercise should be tried. The NCEP guidelines recommend obtaining a lipoprotein profile in women aged over 55 years who have a total cholesterol over 200 mg/dL. As for secondary prevention, trials which have included women have shown at least as much benefit in females, if not more than in men. Women with clinical CAD – regardless of age – should be screened and treated with the same degree of aggressive lipid-lowering therapy as men. Recently, the ACC/AHA consensus panel on the guide to preventive cardiology for women have recommended aggressive targets for LDL-C lowering. A lower optimal triglyceride level of ≤150 mg/dL and an HDL-C ≥45 mg/dL are also emphasized.[39A]

Diabetes mellitus

Patients with diabetes mellitus have a two- to six-fold increase in the risk of CAD, peripheral vascular disease, and cerebrovascular disease.[40] In particular, diabetes is an important risk factor for women.[41] The relative protection from CHD which is seen in premenopausal, non-diabetic women is not observed in diabetic women. In addition to the specific impact of diabetes itself, associated risk factors such as low levels of HDL-C, high triglycerides, and hypertension are found in high prevalence. These risk factors further increase the overall risk for future cardiovascular complications.

As a result of the high CHD risk, the American Diabetes Association (ADA) has published guidelines for screening and monitoring lipoprotein levels in diabetics. The ADA guidelines are in close agreement with those of the NCEP. Aggressive screening and management of lipoprotein abnormalities are recommended. All adult diabetics should have a full lipoprotein analysis, including total cholesterol, triglycerides, HDL-C, and measurement of LDL-C. New guidelines are quite aggressive; for diabetic patients without evidence of CHD, LDL-C levels <100 mg/dL should be the goal, along with vigorous reduction of the other risk factors. These guidelines apply to both men and women. In patients with established CHD or other atherosclerotic disease, the LDL-C goal should also be <100 mg/dL, and as low as feasible. To the extent possible, triglycerides should also be lowered to desirable levels, as these are often the more dense, atherogenic particles which appear to account for at least some of the excessively high risk seen in hypertriglyceridemic diabetic patients.[42] The use of a fibrate (e.g. gemfibrozil) is indicated in insulin-resistant, prediabetic patients, or in subjects with overt diabetes who have the typical diabetic lipid profile of low HDL, high triglyceride, and normal LDL. The results of the VA-HIT study confirmed the efficiency of this approach.[42A] However, when LDL is elevated in a diabetic, fibrate use should be the first line of attack of therapy, usually with a statin.

Table 6.2 *Treatment decisions based on LDL-cholesterol (LDL-C) levels in adults with diabetes (adapted from Diabetes Care[42])*

	Medical nutrition therapy		Drug therapy	
	Initiation level	LDL–C goal	Initiation level	LDL–C goal
With CHD, PVD or CVD	>100	≤100	>100	≤100
Without CHD, PVD and CVD	>100	≤100	≥130[a]	≤100

Values are mg/dL.
[a]For diabetic patients with one or more CHD risk factors [low HDL (<35 mg/dL), hypertension, smoking, family history of cardiovascular disease or microalbuminuria or proteinuria), some authorities recommend an LDL goal of ≤100 mg/dL.
Caveats:
1. Medical nutrition therapy should be attempted before starting pharmacological therapy.
2. Since diabetic men and women are considered to have equal CHD risk, age and sex are not considered as 'risk factors.'
PVD: peripheral vascular disease.

African-Americans

Since 1980, CAD rates have declined faster in whites than in blacks. In addition, sudden cardiac death is much more common among blacks and underscores the need for a prevention strategy.[43] In 1993, death rates from cardiovascular diseases were 47 percent higher for black males than for white males, and 69 percent higher for black females than for white. While modifiable risk factors (e.g. hypertension, smoking, obesity and physical inactivity) are more prevalent among blacks, cholesterol levels are similar to those in whites. Increased Lp(a) has been reported among blacks, but its relationship to CAD is not clear. Because of the high risk – which is particularly concentrated among those in the lower socioeconomic strata – standard lipid screening should be routinely conducted, and aggressive lipid-lowering strategy should be a major part of both primary and secondary prevention strategies in the African-American population.

Asian Indians

An increased prevalence of CAD in Asian Indians both from the native country and the immigrant population has been known for some time. More than 1 million Asian Indians live in the United States, and 1.5 million in the United Kingdom. A disturbing trend has been seen during the past two decades. In the UK, overall coronary mortality declined by 5 percent in men and 1 percent in women, whereas among Asians in the UK, it increased by 6 percent in men and 13 percent in women.[44] Established risk factors such as plasma total cholesterol, hypertension, and smoking do not explain the higher mortality, but there is a higher prevalence of non-insulin-dependent diabetes mellitus, lower plasma HDL-C and higher triglyceride concentrations which contribute to the atherogenic milieu. Insulin resistance has been suggested in Asian Indians as the underlying mechanism leading to the high prevalence of lipid disorders and overall mortality. The data are consistent with the atherogenic lipid profile described earlier,[45] and Asian Indians also have high levels of Lp(a). It is recommended that aggressive screening and an appropriate lipid-lowering strategy be implemented for Asian Indians who are at high risk.

Mexican Americans

On the basis of their cardiovascular risk profile, Mexican Americans are at high risk for CHD. Compared with non-Hispanic whites, Hispanics have a three-fold higher prevalence of diabetes, higher triglyceride levels, more obesity, and lower HDL-C levels. Despite the high levels of cardiovascular risk factors, mortality studies have documented a 15–36 percent lower cardiovascular mortality in Hispanics as compared with non-Hispanic white men.[46] There is no significant difference in total cholesterol levels between Hispanics and non-Hispanic white men. Low Lp(a) may account for reduced cardiovascular risk in this segment of population. Because of the high prevalence of these treatable risk factors, routine screening and appropriate therapy are recommended as part of a prevention strategy.

Native American Indians

Coronary heart disease is the leading cause of death among Native American Indians. The prevalence of CHD varies however, and is lower in Arizona compared with communities in Oklahoma and the Dakotas. The Strong Heart Study found CHD in Native American Indians to be significantly and independently related to age, diabetes, hypertension, obesity, smoking, insulin resistance and low HDL-C.[47] Owing to the rising incidence of CHD in this segment of the population, early screening for the presence of risk factors and aggressive treatment are recommended.

REFERENCES

1. *Heart and Stroke Facts: 1995 Statistical Supplement.* American Heart Association, Dallas, Texas.
2. Johnson CL, Rifkind BM, Sempos CT, *et al.* Declining serum cholesterol levels among U.S. adults. *JAMA* 1993; **269**: 3002–8.
3. Goldman L, Cook EF. The decline in ischemic heart disease mortality rates: an analysis of the comparative effects of medical interventions and changes in lifestyles. *Ann Intern Med* 1984; **101**: 1422–7.
4. National Cholesterol Education Program. *The Second Report of the Expert Panel on Detection, Evaluation and Treatment of High Blood Cholesterol in Adults* (Adult Treatment Panel II), Bethesda, MD; National Institutes of Health, 1993.
5. Guidelines for using serum cholesterol. High density lipoprotein cholesterol and triglyceride levels as screening tests for preventing coronary heart disease in adults. American College of Physicians. *Ann Intern Med* 1996; **124**: 525–17.
6. Canadian Task Force on the Periodic Health Examination. Periodic Health Examination, 1993 Update 2. Lowering the blood cholesterol level to prevent coronary heart disease. *Can Med Assoc J* 1993; **148**: 521–38.
7. Wood D, DeBacker G, Graham I, *et al.* Prevention of coronary heart disease in clinical practice: recommendations of the Task Force of the European Society of Cardiology, European Atherosclerotic Society and European Society of Hypertension. *Eur Heart J* 1998; **19**: 1434–503.
8. Anderson KM, Wilson PWF, Odell PM, *et al.* An updated coronary risk profile: a statement for health professionals. *Circulation* 1991; **83**: 356–62.
9. Sempos CT, Cleeman JI, Carroll MD. Prevalence of high blood cholesterol among US adults: an update based on guidelines from the second report of the National Cholesterol Education Program Adult Treatment Panel. *JAMA* 1993; **269**: 3009–14.
10. Gerber AM, Browner WS, Hulley SB. Cholesterol screening in asymptomatic adults, revisited. *Ann Intern Med* 1996; **124**: 518–31.
11. Shephard J, Cobbe SM, Ford I, *et al.* Prevention of coronary heart disease with Pravastatin in men with hypercholesterolemia. *N Engl J Med* 1995; **333**: 1308–17.
11A. Downs JR, Clearfield M, Weis S, *et al.* Primary prevention of acute coronary events with lovastatin in men and women with average cholesterol levels – results of AFCAPS/TexCAPS study. *JAMA* 1998; **279**: 1615–22.
12. Friedewald WT, Levy RI, Fredricson DS. Estimation of the concentration of low density lipoprotein cholesterol in plasma, without use of preparative ultracentrifugation. *Clin Chem* 1972; **18**: 499–502.
13. McNamara JR, Cohn JS, Wilson PWF, *et al.* Calculated values for low density lipoprotein cholesterol in the assessment of lipid abnormalities and coronary disease risk. *Clin Chem* 1990; **36**: 36–42.
14. Martin MJ, Hulley SB, Browner WS, *et al.* Serum cholesterol, blood pressure and mortality: implications from a cohort of 351,662 men. *Lancet* 1986; **2**: 933–9.

15. LaRosa JC, Hunninghake D, Bush D, *et al.* The cholesterol facts: a summary of the evidence relating dietary fats, serum cholesterol and coronary heart disease: a joint statement by the American Heart Association and the National Heart, Lung and Blood Institute. *Circulation* 1990; **89**: 1721–33.

16. Lipid Research Clinics Coronary Primary Prevention Trial Results II. The relationship of reduction incidence of coronary heart disease to cholesterol lowering. *JAMA* 1984; **251**: 365–74.

17. Muldoon MF, Manuck SB, Matthews KA. Lowering cholesterol concentration and mortality: a quantitative review of primary prevention trials. *Br Med J* 1990; **301**: 309–14.

18. Davis CE, Rykinal BM, Brenner H, *et al.* A single cholesterol measurement underestimates the risk of coronary heart disease. *JAMA* 1990; **264**: 3044–6.

19. Gould AL, Rossouw JW, Santanello NC, *et al.* Cholesterol reduction yields clinical benefit: a new look at old data. *Circulation* 1995; **91**: 2274–82.

20. Kannel WB, Sorlie P, McNamara PM. Prognosis after initial myocardial infarction: The Framingham Study. *Am J Cardiol* 1979; **44**: 53.

21. Schlant RC, Forman S, Stamler J, *et al.* The natural history of coronary disease: prognostic factors after recovery from myocardial infarction in 2789 men: the five year findings of coronary drug project. *Circulation* 1982; **66**: 401.

22. Rothrock JF, Heart RG. Antithrombotic therapy in cerebrovascular disease. *Ann Intern Med* 1991; **115**: 885.

23. Scandinavian Simvastatin Survival Study Group. Randomized trial of cholesterol lowering in 444 patients with coronary heart disease. The Scandinavian Simvastatin Survival Study (4S). *Lancet* 1994; **344**: 1383–9.

24. The Post Coronary Artery Bypass Graft Trial Investigators. The effect of aggressive lowering of low density lipoprotein cholesterol levels and low dose anticoagulation on obstructive changes in saphenous vein coronary artery bypass grafts. *N Engl J Med* 1997; **336**: 153–62.

25. Sacks FM, Pfeffer MA, Moye LA, *et al.* The effect of pravastatin on coronary events after myocardial infarction in patients with average cholesterol levels. *N Engl J Med* 1996; **335**: 1001–9.

26. Superko HR. Beyond LDL cholesterol reduction. *Circulation* 1996; **96**: 2351–4.

27. Superko HR. New aspects of cardiovascular risk factors including small, dense LDL, homocysteinemia and Lp(a). *Curr Opin Cardiol* 1995; **10**: 347–54.

28. Rader DJ, Hoeg JM, Brewer B, Jr. Quantification of plasma apolipoproteins in the primary and secondary prevention of coronary artery disease. *Ann Intern Med* 1994; **120**: 1012–25.

29. Gardner CD, Fortmann SP, Krauss RM. Small low density lipoprotein particles are associated with the incidence of coronary artery disease in men and women. *JAMA* 1996; **276**: 875–81.

30. Stampfer MJ, Krauss RM, Blanche PJ, *et al.* A prospective study of triglyceride level, low density lipoprotein particle diameter and risk of myocardial infarction. *JAMA* 1996; **276**: 882–8.

31. Lamarche B, Tchesnof A, Moorjani S, *et al.* Small, dense low density lipoprotein particles as a predictor of risk of ischemic heart disease in men: prospective results from Quebec Cardiovascular Study. *Circulation* 1997; **95**: 69–73.

32. Boerwinkle E, Leffert CC, Lin J, *et al.* Apolipoprotein (a) gene accounts for greater than 90 percent of variation in plasma lipoprotein (a) concentrations. *J Clin Invest* 1992; **90**: 52–60.

33. Maer EL, Jacobson DW, Robinson K. Homocysteine and coronary atherosclerosis. *J Am Coll Cardiol* 1996; **27**: 517.

34. Clarke R, Daby L, Robinson K, *et al.* Hyperhomocysteinemia: an independent risk factor for vascular disease. *N Engl J Med* 1991; **324**: 1149.
35. Stampfer MJ, Mahrow MR, Willett WC. A prospective study of plasma homocysteine and risk of myocardial infarction in US physicians. *JAMA* 1992; **268**: 877.
36. Arnesen E, Refsun H, Bonaa KH, *et al.* Serum total homocysteine and coronary heart disease. *Int J Epidemiol* 1995; **24**: 704–9.
37. Kannel WB, Wilson WF, *et al.* Update on hyperlipidemia in the elderly: is this a risk factor for heart disease. *Am J Geriatr Cardiol* 1996; **5**: 9–14.
38. Rubin SM, Sidney S, Black DM, *et al.* High blood cholesterol in elderly men and the excess risk of coronary heart disease. *Ann Intern Med* 1990; **113**: 916–20.
39. Vital Statistics of the United States, 1985. Vol. II. Mortality part A. National Center for Health Statistics. DHHS Publication No. 88-1101. Public Health Service. Washington, DC, US Government Printing Office, 1988.
39A. Guide to preventive cardiology for women. AHA/ACC Consensus Panel Statement. *Circulation* 1999; **99**: 2480–4.
40. Stamler J, Vaccaro D, Neaton JD. Multiple Risk Factor Intervention Trial Research Group. Diabetes, other risk factors and 12 yr cardiovascular mortality for men screened in the Multiple Risk Factor Intervention Trial. *Diabetes Care* 1993; **15**: 439–44.
41. Krolenwski AS, Wassam JF, Valsaria P, *et al.* Evolving natural history of coronary artery disease in diabetes mellitus. *Am J Med* 1991; **90**(S): 2A–56S.
42. The American Diabetes Association: clinical practice recommendations. *Diabetes Care* 1999; **22** (Suppl. 1): S1–114.
42A. Rubins HB, Robins SJ, Iwane MK, *et al.* Gemfibrozil for the secondary prevention of coronary heart disease in men with low levels of high-density lipoprotein cholesterol. *N Engl J Med* 1999; **341**: 410–18.
43. Lenfant C. Report of the NIHLBI working group on research in coronary heart disease in blacks. *Circulation* 1994; **90**: 1613–23.
44. Balarajan R. Ethnic differences in mortality from ischemic heart disease in England and Wales. *Br Med J* 1991; **302**: 560–4.
45. Dhavan J. Coronary heart disease risks in Asian Indians. *Curr Opin Lipidol* 1996; **7**: 196–8.
46. Mitchell BD, Hazuda HP, Haffner SM, *et al.* Myocardial infarction in Mexican Americans and non-Hispanic whites: the San Antonio Heart Study. *Circulation* 1991; **83**: 45–51.
47. Howard BV, Lee ET, Cowan LD, *et al.* Coronary heart disease prevalence and its relation to risk factors in American Indians. The Strong Heart Study. *Am J Epidemiol* 1995; **142**: 254–68.

7

Role of diet and lifestyle

NEIL J STONE

INTRODUCTION

Diet has traditionally been the cornerstone of the therapeutic approach to lower lipids. The recent introduction into clinical practice of powerful lipid-lowering medications has made it easier for clinicians to reach therapeutic goals. Owing to the time and resource limitations, it would be easy indeed simply to skip over lifestyle change in dealing with the primary and secondary prevention of coronary heart disease (CHD).

LIFESTYLE CHANGES

There are numerous reasons to recommend a change in lifestyle change, and details of these are outlined in the following sections.

Reduction in low-density lipoprotein (LDL)-cholesterol[1]

Small but meaningful changes in LDL-cholesterol (LDL-C) occur with diets that are lower in saturated fats and dietary cholesterol. As there is great variability seen in the response of human subjects to diets, a dietary trial in each patient is reasonable in order to identify those patients who respond in significant fashion.

This response can occur even if the patient is on medication, as dietary benefits on the lipid panel are often additive to those obtained with medication. Moreover, in four large-scale studies where dietary cholesterol intake was very large, there was a relationship with cardiovascular endpoints that was independent of the serum cholesterol level.

Improvement in risk factors such as hypertension and diabetes[2,3]

A diet which is rich in fruits, vegetables, and low-fat dairy foods and with reduced saturated and total fat can substantially lower blood pressure. The Dietary Approaches to Stop Hypertension (DASH) was a randomized controlled feeding study of 459 adults with systolic blood pressures <160 mmHg and diastolic blood pressures of 80–95 mmHg. The above therapeutic dietary plan, without sodium restriction or weight loss, resulted in significantly lower blood pressure in all subgroups examined. Significant weight gain after the age of 18 years is an important marker for both CHD risk and diabetes,[4] and the prevention of such weight gain should be an important goal in the primary prevention of CHD.

Reduction in high triglycerides and elevation of high–density lipoprotein (HDL)–cholesterol levels[1]

As will be noted later in the chapter, diet and exercise are among the best methods to effect beneficial changes in triglycerides and HDL-cholesterol (HDL-C).

Reduction in coronary endpoints seen in controlled, clinical trials[4–11]

Numerous investigations have been performed over the past 50 years examining diet and CHD endpoints, but most of these trials have been flawed by design problems. A sample of informative studies is provided below. The Oslo dietary and smoking intervention trial examined the effects of dietary change and smoking cessation on CHD in hypercholesterolemic men. The intervention group received a diet that was low in saturated fat and also received counseling to reduce smoking. A reduction in serum cholesterol by 10 percent in the intervention group yielded a 47 percent reduction in the incidence of sudden death and myocardial infarction (MI), which contrasted with the control group. At 5 years, the difference in total mortality between the groups reached statistical significance.[5]

Singh and coworkers performed a randomized, single blind, controlled clinical trial in MI survivors. The intervention group had more fruit, vegetables, nuts, and grain products added to the usual post-MI fat-reduced diet.[6] Both groups consumed an almost vegetarian diet, eating eggs four to five times each week and meat once or twice weekly. The intervention group was urged to eat at least 400 g/day of fruits and vegetables. In this small study there was a significant reduction in serum cholesterol, body weight, the incidence of cardiac events, and total mortality.

The Lyon Diet Heart Study was a randomized, controlled trial with survivors of MI that were randomized to an intervention diet that had a Mediterranean style and contrasted with those on a usual care diet.[7] The intervention group was encouraged to eat more bread, vegetables, and fish, and to have fruit at least once daily with less red meat (replaced with poultry) and a special margarine that was made with canola oil and was particularly rich in alpha linolenic acid (a plant-based, omega-3 fatty acid). Only 30 percent of the total cohort group and less than 50 percent of the total experimental group provided dietary data at the conclusion of the study raising questions about the dietary mechanisms responsible for the results that appeared to be independent of change in lipids.[8] The results were so dramatic, however, that corroborative studies should be carried out. Those in the intervention group had a 50–70 percent reduction in recurrent CHD endpoints. It should be noted that the intervention study group followed approximately a 30 percent total fat, 8 percent saturated fat and 200 mg/day dietary cholesterol diet. It was thus very similar to an AHA Step II diet and the therapeutic diet recommended by the Adult Treatment Panel (ATP) III of the National Cholesterol Education Program (NCEP). The control group in the Lyon trial consumed about 34 percent of calories from fat, 12 percent from saturated fat, and consumed slightly more than 300 mg of dietary cholesterol per day.

Studies utilizing serial angiograms to indicate beneficial change with therapy have added further insights. Investigators in the Heidelberg trial restricted total fat to less than 20 percent of calories and prescribed regular and intense physical exercise.[9] Although initial LDL-C reductions obtained on the metabolic ward could not be sustained with the free-living phase over the course of the first year of the trial, the intervention group did show a significant improvement on serial coronary angiograms with less progression and more regression than was seen in the control group. The best metabolic predictors in this study were total cholesterol/HDL-C ratio and the LDL-C.[10]

The St Thomas Atherosclerosis Trial (STARS) contrasted the effects of a low saturated fat diet and/or cholestyramine resin in British men with angina pectoris who underwent serial angiography.[11] The intervention diet restricted total fat to 27 percent of total calories and saturated fat to 8–10 percent of total calories. In addition, the diet was high in fiber, chiefly as pectin. Beneficial effects in coronary luminal change were seen in the intervention groups, with LDL-C as the best predictor of change. Symptoms were also improved in the dietary group.

Further analyses demonstrated higher total fat and saturated fat intake in the usual care group than in the dietary intervention group.[12] Subjects with disease progression consumed 42 g/day of saturated fat, whereas those with regression consumed only 21 g/day. The authors concluded that saturated fat intake significantly influenced the progression of coronary artery disease (CAD), although by mechanisms other than by effects on LDL.

The Stanford Coronary Risk Intervention Project (SCRIP) utilized serial angiography in a 4-year multifactor intervention trial in 300 men and women with CHD.[13] The intervention group underwent multiple interventions, including instruction in a low-fat, low-cholesterol and high-carbohydrate diet with a goal of <20 percent energy from fat, <6 percent from saturated fat, and <75 mg of cholesterol per day. The patients underwent a specific endurance exercise training program, and smokers underwent a supervised stop-smoking program. The evaluation of serial quantitative coronary angiograms showed significant reductions in new lesion formation in the coronary arteries of those randomized to the intervention group. On-study dietary fat intake was the best statistical correlate of new lesion formation. Participants randomized to the risk-reduction group preferentially increased complex carbohydrate intake to offset the reduction in dietary fat restriction. Further analysis suggested that reductions in dietary fat decreased the rate of new lesion formation by mechanisms not limited to LDL reduction.

Ornish and coworkers[14] described a multifactor intervention trial where 28 patients were assigned to an experimental group (low-fat vegetarian diet, smoking cessation, stress management training, and moderate exercise) and 20 to a usual-care control group. The vegetarian-style diet in the intervention group had only 7 percent of total calories from fat. Initial and follow-up studies showed that the intervention group had beneficial changes in symptoms, nuclear perfusion endpoints, and angiographic endpoints as compared to a control group. The small number of subject and problems with randomization in this study limit extrapolation of this regimen to the 'average' patient with CHD.

Reduction in sudden death in those with prior MI

The large intake of marine lipids and low rates of CHD in Greenland Eskimos (Inuit) focused attention on omega-3 fatty acids as a potential useful dietary intervention. Epidemiological studies confirmed that in some – but not all – populations, eating some fish meals per week resulted in lower mortality from CHD. However, a carefully controlled clinical trial showed that fish oil supplementation at 8 g per day does not prevent restenosis after coronary angioplasty.[15] In addition, two trials in which patients with angiographically proven CHD received 6 g of omega-3 fatty acids each day showed either no significant or minimal improvement in angiographic appearance.

The results of several studies have suggested that fish intake can be beneficial to those with heart disease. The Diet and Reinfarction Trial (DART) randomized men to various treatment groups. Those instructed to eat fish had a 29 percent decline in all-cause mortality as compared to those in the placebo group that was independent of the serum cholesterol.[16] A population-based case-control study from Seattle showed that victims of primary cardiac arrest had evidence of lower fish intake than matched controls.[17] Both short[18] and long-term follow-up of the MI survivors in the Lyon Diet Heart Study documented fewer cardiac outcomes, but particularly sudden death in the intervention group as noted above. It is tempting to speculate that the omega-3 fatty acid-rich margarine consumed by the intervention group was important in this finding.

Reduction in the cost of drug therapy[19,20]

Small, but meaningful, reductions in LDL-C with diet can reduce the need for larger and more expensive dosages of medications. Whilst initial dosages of hexamethylglutaryl-coenzyme A (HMG-CoA) reductase inhibitors (statins) lower LDL-C markedly, as the dosage is increased there is a reduction in the amount of

LDL-C lowering with each doubling of the dose. This 'log-dose response' relationship emphasizes the incremental value of diet to statin therapy; LDL lowering with diet is equivalent to a doubling of the statin dose (i.e. another 6–7% of LDL lowering on average).

Lifetime benefits of lifestyle change in shifting the mean cholesterol level of the population[21]

Statisticians calculate that a shift in the mean serum cholesterol level of the population by 10 percent could reduce CHD events by 30 percent. This is achievable with population-based strategies to improve lifestyle.

THERAPEUTIC LIPID–LOWERING DIETS[2]

The NCEP and the American Heart Association (AHA) have for many years advocated a stepwise dietary approach to lower LDL-C. The Step I diet restricted saturated fat to less than 10 percent of calories and dietary cholesterol to <300 mg per day. The Step II diet restricted saturated fat to less than 7 percent of calories and dietary cholesterol to <200 mg/day. The Step I diet is essentially a 'population' diet, and is no longer used clinically as most patients are already on a dietary pattern similar to this. In addition, in the various angiographic intervention studies performed with statins, those on placebo and a Step I diet had documented angiographic progression at the end of the study. The Step II diet or 'high-risk' diet is designed to help patients achieve optimal reduction of LDL-C through diet. It is more rigorous than the Step I diet, and requires individualized dietary counseling. Dietary fat is restricted to less than 30 percent of total calories, and achieving and maintaining a normal body weight is emphasized. The current AHA[22] and NCEP ATP III[23] dietary plans emphasize for LDL lowering approximately 30 percent fat, less than 7 percent total fat, and <200 mg per day of dietary cholesterol. A dietary plan rich in fiber with daily consumption of fruit and vegetables is also advised. The ATP III therapeutic diet (Table 7.1) recommended that total fat intake should not be less than 25 percent or greater than 35 percent of total calories. The reasons for this range were:

- To avoid the problems with low HDL-C, high triglycerides, and decreased adherence when total fat in the diet is restricted to less than 25 percent of total energy.
- To avoid the problems with a higher carbohydrate intake, particularly in diabetics and those with impaired glucose tolerance, an increase in unsaturated fats may be useful and hence total fat intake may exceed 30 percent of total energy (but no more than 35 percent).

ATP III defined the metabolic syndrome as a constellation of symptoms and signs that increase the risk of both diabetes and CHD. Clinical identification requires the identification of three or more of the following:

- Waist circumference >101 cm (40 inches) in men and >89 cm (35 inches) in women
- Triglycerides ≥150 mg/dL
- HDL-C <40 mg/dL in men; <50 mg/dL in women
- Blood pressure ≥130/≥85 mmHg
- Fasting blood glucose ≥110–125 mg/dL

The panel emphasized the importance of regular exercise and weight control in the approach to patients with this syndrome.

Table 7.1 *Diet composition for the therapeutic diet in ATP III*

Nutrient	Recommended intake
Saturated fat[a]	Less than 7% of total calories
Polyunsaturated fat	Up to 10% of total calories
Monounsaturated fat	Up to 20% of total calories
Total fat	25–35% of total calories
Carbohydrate[b]	50–60% of total calories
Fiber	20–30 g per day
Protein	Approximately 15% of total calories
Cholesterol	Less than 200 mg per day
Total calories (energy)[c]	Balance energy intake and expenditure to maintain desirable body weight/prevent weight gain

[a]*Trans* fatty acids are another LDL-raising fat that should be kept at a low intake.
[b]Carbohydrate should be derived predominantly from foods rich in complex carbohydrates, including grains (especially whole grains), fruit and vegetables.
[c]Daily energy expenditure should include at least moderate physical activity (contributing approximately 200 kcal per day).
Source: Executive Summary of the Third Report of the National Cholesterol Education Program (NCEP) Expert Panel on Detection, Evaluation, and Treatment of High Blood Cholesterol in Adults (Adult Treatment Panel III). *JAMA* 2001; 285: 2486–97.

Importance of lowering saturated fat and dietary cholesterol intake

While the media often (in error, I believe) focus on the percentage of calories as total fat, physicians should remind their patients that reduction of food which is rich in saturated fatty acids (SFA) and cholesterol, together with the avoidance of extra calories, to prevent obesity are the hallmarks of a cardioprotective dietary plan. Useful questions by the health professional include asking how often do you eat:

- Animal fats and fried foods?
- High-fat cheeses and dairy products?
- High-fat foods when you eat out?
- Commercial products high in fat and sugars, such as cakes, cookies, ice-cream, candies, or pies?

SFA were shown in a large-scale epidemiological cross-country comparison to explain much of the difference in CHD rates between countries.[24] Metabolic ward studies have shown the powerful effects of SFA in raising LDL-C. A recent multicenter randomized, cross-over-design trial examined the effects of reducing dietary SFA in 103 healthy, free-living adults who ate prepared meals.[25] The results showed that with stepwise reduction of SFA there were parallel reductions in total and LDL-C.

Dietary effects were similar in sub-groups of men and women, and also in blacks. Moreover, reducing total dietary fat without reducing SFA in the diet does not lower total plasma cholesterol.[26] An assessment by questionnaire of a large cohort of health professionals (possibly different than a general population sample) suggested that their low fiber content and associations with other risk factors, at least in part, explain the adverse effects of high saturated fat and cholesterol diets.[27]

Sources of SFA include animal fats, and vegetable sources such as coconut and palm kernel oil. Stearic acid (C18:0), although a SFA, does not appear to raise serum cholesterol levels as it is converted to a monounsaturated fat (oleic acid) in the body. Nonetheless, in the STARS clinical trial, progression of atherosclerotic disease as assessed by serial angiography was directly, strongly and independently associated with intake of SFAs of chain length 14 to 18.[28] This effect was not completely explained by the effects of SFA on raising LDL-C. Even after adjustment, intake of stearic acid, a saturated fat, remained independently predictive of progression.

Dietary cholesterol provokes a lesser and quite variable response in LDL-C in human subjects as contrasted with saturated fat intake. At higher intakes than are seen today, four large epidemiological studies showed a relationship to CHD.[29] One of these investigations, the Western Electric study, showed that dietary cholesterol was related to CHD at all levels of serum cholesterol level.[30]

These dietary plans have had impact on the nation's health. The total fat and SFA intakes as a percentage of total energy have been declining over the past 30 years in the United States.[31] Yet many patients do not eat a good diet and a large body of nutritional data is developing that suggest beneficial modifications to these plans.

Biological and clinical variables that affect dietary responses

These variables can be assigned to four groups:

GENETIC

Knowledge of apolipoprotein E phenotype or LDL sub-class, for example, can predict responses to diet.

CLINICAL

1. Body weight: patients with abdominal obesity and signs of insulin resistance or metabolic syndrome should be viewed differently from those who do not have this attribute.
2. Changes in body weight with diet: it is important to assess lipid responses to diet once the individual has attained a stable weight for at least 3 weeks. Lipid changes may be exacerbated during weight gain and may be markedly better during weight loss.

LIPID STATUS

1. Those with combined high levels of cholesterol and triglycerides (above the 75th percentile) respond differently in feeding experiments than those with high cholesterol only.
2. Baseline lipid status: the higher the serum cholesterol or triglycerides, the greater the average response to diet.
3. Lipid pattern: those patients with very high triglyceride levels (>1000 mg/dL) are very sensitive to weight loss, total dietary fat restriction and use of fish oils. Individuals with very high triglycerides are prone to pancreatitis and total fat *must* be severely restricted, and the high triglycerides lowered by a combination of lifestyle change and medications such as fibrates or niacin.

COMPLIANCE STATUS

1. Many patients given therapeutic diets are non-compliant.
2. Those who receive individualized instruction, become aware of external limitations and get regular feedback, may be in a better position to achieve success.

Controversies in diet

Physicians need to understand current trends in the literature regarding dietary therapy as patient's turn to physicians for advice! Several types of dietary pattern are advocated, and the arguments for these are as follows:

1. The diet should be low in total fat (as well as SFA) and increased in complex carbohydrate. Proponents argue that:[32]
- A low-fat diet lowers post-prandial lipid levels.
- Lower-fat diets encourage weight loss – a lower energy cost for carbohydrate as compared with fat.
- Lower-fat diets may reduce the incidence of certain cancers (e.g. breast, colon, prostate).
- Increased dietary fiber is beneficial.
- Increased carbohydrate does not mean a dietary increase in sugars and sweeteners.

Comment: The combination of low dietary SFA and cholesterol with an increase in dietary fiber has been the 'backbone' of the AHA diets for several decades. A major problem has been the increased consumption of 'no-fat' foods laden with sweeteners.

2. The diet should utilize monounsaturated fats to replace SFA and avoid an excessive amount of complex carbohydrates. Proponents argue that:[33]
- High-carbohydrate diets lower HDL-C.
- Very low-fat, high-carbohydrate diets worsen the lipid abnormalities seen with insulin resistance and may promote formation of small, dense LDL.
- Fat restriction does not prevent obesity.
- Evidence relating to fat and cancer is not as simple as it seems.

- Fat intake has no overall relation to breast cancer.
- Red meat, not total fat, relates to colon cancer.
- Animal, not vegetable, fat relates to prostate cancer.
- Diets high in monounsaturated fats (the Mediterranean experience) can be associated with longevity and low rates of CHD and cancer.

Comment: This type of diet may be particularly beneficial in diabetics. The higher monounsaturated fatty acid intake and the lower carbohydrate intake may lead to higher levels of HDL-C. An important caveat is to avoid extra calories which might lead to obesity.

3. Evidence supports a 'Mediterranean-style' diet as given in the Lyon trial.[7] In this trial, subjects consumed a diet low in SFA and dietary cholesterol, but sources of omega-3 fatty acids were emphasized, with a lower intake of omega-6 fatty acids. Proponents argue that:[34]
- A simple change in diet, independent of effects on cholesterol, may have a profound change in cardiovascular event rates of MI survivors.
- The continued high adherence rate to the dietary regimen over 46 months.
- Omega-3 fatty acids have been disappearing from our diet in favor of omega-6 fatty acids.
- Animal studies have reported potent anti-arrhythmic effects of long-chain polyunsaturated fatty acids of the n-3 class, and secondary prevention trials have shown a significant effect on reduction of sudden death (see above).

Comment: In the Lyon trial, the intervention group had an increase in omega-3 fatty acids by emphasizing an increase in sources of linolenic acid. Longer chain sources of omega-3 fatty acids are also found in cold-water fish. The case for increasing omega-3 fatty acids is much stronger for secondary prevention (and particularly those at risk for sudden death) than for primary prevention. Issues particularly pertinent for recommending increased omega-3 fatty acids as increased fish intake for primary prevention include:

- Decreased cell-mediated immunity when the Step II diet was supplemented with a high fish intake as compared to that seen with a diet low in fish intake (121–188 g versus 33 g fish per day).[35]
- Problems with obtaining fish in various parts of the country.
- Concerns about mercury toxicity attenuating the benefit seen with fish intake.[36]
- Inconsistent relationship between fish intake and the primary prevention of CHD.

4. Some advocate a very low fat diet. This has been defined as a diet with the following characteristics:[37]
- 15 percent or less of total calories are derived from fat (33 g for a 2000-calorie diet).
- Fat calories distributed approximately equally among saturated, monounsaturated, and polyunsaturated sources.
- Approximately 15 percent of total daily calories consumed from protein sources.
- Approximately 70 percent of total daily calories consumed from carbohydrates.

Comments: Although several small studies of very low-fat diets and CHD have been reported in the literature, the data from the Lifestyle Heart Trial[14] have generated renewed interest in this approach. This intervention trial used a *very* low level of dietary fat (7% of calories). Despite beneficial cardiovascular effects seen in this trial, the small size, problems with randomization and lack of larger-scale supporting trial data make it difficult to generalize the Lifestyle Heart Trial results to the general population. Other concerns regarding a very low-fat diet include nutritional considerations (knowledgeable selection of sources of essential fatty acids and unresolved questions regarding the feasibility of long-term restriction of certain foods) and the effects on triglycerides and HDL-C levels. The AHA advised that, pending further data, 'a limited group of motivated, high-risk persons with elevated LDL-C levels and/or preexisting cardiovascular disease may benefit from very low fat diets but only with support, careful supervision, and regular follow-up by the healthcare provider.'

DIETARY COMPONENTS THAT INFLUENCE LIPIDS, RISK FACTORS AND CHD

Finally, it is important to consider the effect on risk factors and CHD of components of the diet. A brief assessment of some of the factors is given below.

Trans fatty acids (TFA)

Elaidic acid, the *trans* isomer of oleic acid, is the most common example of TFA. Partial hydrogenation converts the naturally occurring *cis* double bonds which keep the fat liquid at room temperature to the straighter *trans* isomers that are more tightly packed and keep the fat solid at room temperature. The following facts are worth noting about TFA:

- Sources include stick margarine and shortening, milk, butter, cheese and commercially processed baked good. TFA have replaced the highly saturated tropical oils in certain foods.
- At low levels of intake, TFA raise LDL-C less than saturated fats and do not raise HDL-C. At high levels of intake, TFA raise LDL-C and lower HDL-C.
- In two large observational trials, intake of TFA correlated with the incidence of CHD.

Conclusion: Both saturated fats and TFA should be reduced in the diet and kept under 10 percent of total calories.

Omega-6 polyunsaturated fatty acids

Polyunsaturated fatty acids (PUFA) include omega-3 and omega-6 fatty acids. The convention is to name the unsaturated fatty acids after the number of the carbon atom where the first double bond appears from the terminal end of the carbon chain. Important facts about omega-6 PUFA are:

- Sources of omega-6 PUFA include linoleic acid (an essential fatty acid that cannot be synthesized by the body) which is present in seed oils such as safflower oil, cottonseed oil, and corn oil.
- Metabolic ward studies showed that PUFA were half as potent in lowering serum cholesterol as SFA were in raising them.
- One clinical trial with a high omega-6 PUFA diet demonstrated an increased risk for cholelithiasis.
- Concerns exist from experimental studies about cancer risk at high levels of omega-6 PUFA intake (over 10%).

Conclusion: Although omega-6 PUFA are essential fatty acids, very high intakes (above 10%) should be avoided as it is not clear that the benefits exceed the risks.

Omega-3 PUFA

Omega-3 fatty acids may be of either plant-based or marine origin. There is increasing emphasis on recommending these for cardiac patients. Plant-based omega-3 fatty acids include alpha linolenic acid found in tofu, soybean, and canola oil and nuts. Marine-based omega-3 fatty acids include eicosapentaenoic acid (EPA) and docosahexenoic acid (DHA); these are found in fatty fish such as salmon and mackerel. DHA may be particularly important for cardioprotective effects.

Although marine lipids reduce triglycerides and may be useful as therapeutic adjuncts in those patients with very high levels of triglycerides, this effect may not be totally responsible for the cardioprotective effects. Other potentially beneficial effects include reduced platelet aggregation and prolonged bleeding times. A systematic review of studies based on individual records of fish or n-3 PUFA intake and CHD death concluded that fish intake was not associated with reduction in CHD risk in low-risk populations, although benefit was seen in higher-risk populations.[38] The results of several studies have supported the contention that diets rich in omega-3 PUFA are beneficial in patients with CHD.[6,7,16] Moreover, in the large multi-center GISSI prevention study that followed male and female survivors of MI, those randomized to fish oil capsules, but not to vitamin E (300 mg/day) had reduced subsequent cardiovascular rates (fatal and non-fatal MI and stroke).[39]

Conclusion: Fish may be a good source of protein that is low in SFA. Patients should try to eat two fish meals (not fried and without high-fat sauces) per week, and also consider sources of alpha linolenic acid in the diet, such as canola and flaxseed oils. Fish oil capsules as used in GISSI[39] and DART[16] trials should be considered for those patients who have had an MI and are at risk for sudden death. Further studies may be useful in those patients who cannot obtain or tolerate marine sources of omega-3 PUFA and who are at increased risk of sudden death. Recent data support this dietary approach as a means of decreasing sudden cardiac death.

Dietary fiber[40]

Fiber is non-digestible, plant-based carbohydrate. Currently, the average fiber intake in the United States is about 15 mg per day, or about one-half of the recommended amount. The new ATP III therapeutic diet suggests increased dietary fiber and plant sterols (see below) as dietary adjuncts that can further reduce LDL-C levels. Important facts about dietary fiber include:

- Sources of viscous (previously called soluble) fiber include: dried beans, oat products, fruits, vegetables, and grains (pectins, guar gums and mucilages).
- The gradual increase in viscous fiber will further lower LDL-C.
- Populations with increased fiber intake show reduced risk of both MI and stroke.

Conclusion: Increase total dietary fiber to 25–30 g per day.

Plant sterols[41]

ATP III further suggested the ingestion of plant sterol/stanols. In general, humans ingest almost as much plant sterols (vegetarians have more) as they do dietary cholesterol. In fact, sterols such as beta sitosterol have been used since the 1950s to reduce blood cholesterol.

- Plant sterols are poorly absorbed (stanols even less), and reduce blood cholesterol levels by reducing the micellar absorption of dietary and biliary cholesterol.
- Margarines using plant sterol or stanol esters can lower LDL-C in dose-related fashion up to 14 percent. HDL-C levels are unchanged. There is an LDL-C effect that is additive to that obtained with statins. Interestingly, older subjects may have a greater response than younger subjects.
- Plant sterol/stanol ester margarines do not cause fat malabsorption. No significant side effects have been reported.
- Since there is a concern about lower beta-carotene levels in some studies, they should not be used in pregnant women and children, but used as adjuncts for the treatment of hypercholesterolemia. One exception would be children with familial hypercholesterolemia.

Conclusion: The use of plant sterols and stanols in margarines and salad dressings can be useful adjuncts for additional LDL-C lowering. This may permit LDL C goals to be attained and forestall use of medications or reduce the total statin dose required to reach LDL-C goals.

Soy protein

Soy has been used for a long time, and is a vegetable protein found in soy milk, tofu, and tempeh.
   It is a rich source of dietary phytoestrogens.

- Studies of soy protein in hypercholesterolemic subjects show that lower levels of LDL-C are obtained, but HDL-C levels are unchanged.
- Isoflavones appear to be important for these effects.

Conclusion: Further studies are needed to document any cardiovascular benefit of soy. The use of vegetable protein to replace animal protein, with its associated saturated fat, is consistent with current dietary guidelines.

Alcohol[42]

Intake of alcohol increases triglycerides by increasing the synthesis of the very low-density lipoproteins (VLDL). Thus, alcohol can aggravate hypertriglyceridemia. In patients with genetic hypertriglyceridemia, excess alcohol intake and fat can provoke the chylomicronemia syndrome and pancreatitis. Beneficial effects of alcohol include:

- Alcohol raises HDL-C. The effects on HDL-C appear to account for at least half of the observed benefit of alcohol on CHD risk.[43]
- Alcohol also has beneficial effects on fibrinolytic activity.
- There is an inverse association between alcohol usage and CHD. Observational data suggest that there is no advantage to red wine, white wine or beer, and that the major cardiovascular benefit derives from the alcohol rather than the other components of each type of drink.[44]
- Despite some studies looking at components of red wine and factors that increase CHD risk, the benefits of red over white wine remain unproven. Interestingly, the increased consumption of alcohol in France (and red wine in particular) explains little of the difference between CHD rates in Britain and France.[45]
- Moderate to severe alcohol consumption can affect left ventricular function (women have cardiomyopathy from excess usage at a lower total cumulative dose than men), trigger atrial fibrillation, raise blood pressure, and increase stroke rates.

Conclusion: Alcohol cannot be recommended generally for cardiovascular health due to its adverse effects at higher dosage.

BEHAVIORAL MEASURES TO RAISE HDL–CHOLESTEROL[46]

Behavioral measures to raise HDL-C should always be considered when a higher HDL-C is sought. These include:

- Weight reduction.
- Less carbohydrate in the diet. In particular, a lower intake of food of high glycemic index, notably pasta, oats, whole grain products, vegetables, and whole fruit. Dietary carbohydrates with a high glycemic index cause high post-prandial glucose and an insulin response.
- Cessation of cigarette smoking.
- Aerobic exercise; this may be particularly useful in those patients in whom lower fat intakes reduce HDL-C.

A carefully controlled clinical trial demonstrated significantly more weight loss with diet and exercise together than diet alone. Moreover, this loss was primarily fat weight and resulted in a greater improvement in the waist-to-hip ratio in both men and women. In women, the ratio was not reduced in those who underwent diet alone.[47] Changes in HDL-C with exercise do not occur quickly; it may take between

4 months and 1 year of regular exercise before significant changes in HDL-C are seen.[48]

Exercise also helps to lower triglycerides. The results of metabolic studies suggest that aerobic exercise helps to lower fasting and post-prandial triglyceride values, even when body weight is maintained

Anti-oxidants[49]

During the past decade, physicians have noted that increasing numbers of patients took vitamin supplements in the hope that this would reduce the risk of CHD. However, despite intriguing observational data suggesting benefit from anti-oxidants, clinical trial data – much like that seen with estrogens and CHD – have not substantiated the benefit.

Alpha tocopherol (vitamin E)

Alpha tocopherol is a potent lipid-soluble anti-oxidant that is carried on LDL, and has the following characteristics:

- Food sources include seed oils, nuts, avocados, whole grain and fortified cereals, eggs, and green vegetables.
- Vitamin E ingested from the diet varies inversely with risk of CHD death in postmenopausal women from Iowa.[50] The results of a recent study showed that nurses who consumed nuts had a reduced risk of fatal and non-fatal MI.[51] Obtaining vitamin E from the diet may be a useful primary prevention strategy for CHD.
- A randomized, double-blind clinical trial of subjects with angiographically proven CHD – the Cambridge Heart Antioxidant Trial (CHAOS) – showed that those patients given vitamin E (a natural source was used in this trial) had a significant reduction in non-fatal MI rates after 1 year as compared with placebo.[52] There was no significant reduction in total mortality, however.
- Two large clinical trials did not show benefit. The Heart Outcomes Prevention Evaluation Study (HOPE) trial also showed no benefit from vitamin E supplementation. In this trial, which had a 2×2 factorial design, ramipril did show benefit versus placebo.[50] The GISSI prevention study in survivors of MI (see above) also did not identify, for vitamin E supplementation, any significant beneficial effect on the primary endpoints of the study.[39]
- In a large clinical trial – the Heart Protection Study – those randomized to vitamin E had no difference in event rates for CHD and total mortality compared with those receiving placebo.[54]
- In a 3-year angiographic trial of CHD subjects with low HDL-C, those randomized to simvastatin and niacin showed evidence for regression on serial angiography. A surprising result occurred when anti-oxidant vitamins (vitamin E, beta carotene, vitamin C, and selenium) were added to the lipid-lowering regimen. This caused lower HDL-C levels and progression on serial angiography, which contrasted with the regression seen when simvastatin and niacin were given without vitamins.[55]

Conclusion: Now, after three large, well-constructed clinical trials have shown no significant effect on the primary cardiovascular endpoint and without any significant effect on total mortality, the evidence for using vitamin E in the secondary prevention of CHD is weak at best. In those patients with low HDL-C, megavitamins appear to decrease the benefit of lipid-lowering therapy and cannot be recommended for the secondary prevention of CHD.

Beta carotene[56–58]

Beta carotene is a vitamin A precursor which is lipid-soluble and has the following characteristics:

- It is a weak anti-oxidant.
- Food sources include carrots or green leafy vegetables such as broccoli.
- Three randomized clinical trials using beta carotene supplementation showed no beneficial effects on cancer or cardiovascular disease.
- Beta carotene supplementation provides an adverse effect on lung cancer and the risk of death from lung cancer, cardiovascular disease, and from all causes in cigarette smokers and workers exposed to asbestos.

Conclusion: There is no indication for beta-carotene supplements in the primary or secondary prevention of cardiovascular disease. They may cause harm.

Vitamin C

Vitamin C is a water-soluble anti-oxidant that is widely available in fruits and vegetables. Deficiencies of this vitamin cause scurvy.

Conclusion: No clinical trial data are available to support the routine use of vitamin C.

Flavonoids

Flavonoids are strong anti-oxidants that are found in vegetables, fruits, and beverages such as tea and wine. Observational studies have shown that flavonoid intake was significantly inversely associated with mortality from CHD, although its effect was small when compared with that of SFA.

Homocyst(e)ine, folic acid, and vitamins B_6 and B_{12}[59]

Homocysteine is a sulfur-containing amino acid that results from the demethylation of methionine. It is rapidly oxidized in plasma to two disulfides. Plasma/serum total homocysteine is termed homocyst(e)ine, which is the sum of all three components.

- Plasma homocyst(e)ine levels exhibit a strong inverse association with plasma folate.[60] Sources of folate in the diet (as well as B_{12} and B_6) include vegetables, fruits, legumes, meats, fish, and fortified grains and cereals.

- Vitamin supplementation with folic acid can lower raised homocyst(e)ine levels. Daily intake of 400 mg of folic acid and 3 mg of vitamin B_6 was correlated with the lowest risk of CHD in a 14-year follow-up study of a large cohort of women.[61]
- Moderate elevations of homocyst(e)ine are estimated to occur in up to 50 percent of patients with coronary, cerebral, or peripheral arterial occlusive diseases. Not all prospective studies, however, have documented a relationship between plasma homocyst(e)ine and cardiovascular disease.
- In those patients who have undergone percutaneous coronary interventions (PCI) with either balloon and/or stent, the use of folic acid (1 mg), B_{12} (500 mg), and vitamin B_6 (10 mg) per day significantly increased the minimal lumen diameter, and was associated with a lower rate of restenosis in the target lesion.[62] None the less, these data await corroboration by other investigations.
- At levels above 1 mg/day of folic acid, vitamin B_{12} toxicity may be masked. Supplementation with folic acid should be avoided in the elderly and anorectic patients without first investigating B_{12} status. Vitamins B_{12} and B_6 supplementation may further lower homocyst(e)ine levels.
- Potential mechanisms for the increased risk of CHD and stroke include deleterious effects on endothelial function, platelet adhesiveness, thrombotic tendency, and smooth muscle cells

Conclusion: Population-wide screening for homocyst(e)ine excess is not warranted. A high-risk strategy would include screening for those with a personal or family history of premature cardiovascular disease or with conditions known to be associated with higher levels of homocysteine, such as renal failure or use of nicotinic acid. It is reasonable for those patients with higher levels of homocyst(e)ine to increase their intake of vitamin-fortified foods and to consider the daily use of supplements of folic acid, vitamin B_6 and vitamin B_{12}. In those patients undergoing PCI – particularly balloon angioplasty – a combination of folic acid, B_6, and pyridoxine should not be given routinely until more studies are available.

Fad diets

There likely will always be dietary fads that capture the public's imagination and for which physicians are expected to have a ready response. Although this chapter has tried to provide some of the evidence that supports the diets proposed by the AHA and the NCEP, a few words about alternative dietary plans are in order. As a rough approximation, most dietary alternatives involve changes in carbohydrates and fats. The two most well known are the low-fat, high-carbohydrate diets and the high-fat, low-carbohydrate diets.

Previously, Ornish and colleagues (see above) popularized a very low-fat, high complex carbohydrate dietary plan associated with other preventive measures such as exercise, stress reduction, and smoking cessation. The concerns with his dietary plan have been compliance, nutrient deficiency, and lack of additional evidence supporting this recommendation over those proposed by the AHA and the NCEP. Compliance is a problem for those who are not exceptionally motivated because of the difficulty in eating such a high-volume diet (foods on this diet are not energy dense and hence the volume of food is much greater). Some concern has also been expressed regarding essential fatty acid deficiencies if fat restriction were too extreme.

On the other hand, the increase in obesity in western countries is particularly alarming. Advocates of a high-fat (and hence high-protein) diet with little or no carbohydrate can point to a diet that satisfies the appetite and causes, in the short term, weight loss. Weight is lost because these diets are hypocaloric. Often, however, the low carbohydrate intake causes a water diuresis and so when carbohydrate is again consumed, water is also retained. Diets high in protein are particularly worrisome for diabetics and other patients with renal problems. Although lipids may be improved in the short term (there is a short-term benefit from weight loss), in the long term the patients have not learned healthful dietary habits as regards restricting saturated fatty acids in the diet. Moreover, there are essentially no scientific data available to support the efficacy of these diets long term. In contrast to the poor adherence long-term seen with the low carbohydrate diets, a recent clinical trial of 522 middle-aged, overweight subjects with impaired glucose tolerance demonstrated the benefit of a modest weight reduction of 5 percent or more, a total fat intake of 30 percent or less, a saturated fat intake of 10 percent or less, an increase of fiber to 15 g per 1000 kcal/day, and moderate exercise for at least 30 min per day.[63]

After slightly more than 3 years, this lifestyle change reduced the incidence of diabetes by 58 percent. The diet consisted of frequent ingestion of whole-grain products, vegetables, fruits, low-fat milk and meat products, soft margarines, and vegetable oils rich in monounsaturated fatty acids.

Compliance

Most clinicians recognize that many patients do not exhibit long-term adherence to lifestyle-modification. Others have commented that 43 percent of patients do not follow long-term regimens – even for the treatment of life-threatening diseases – and 75 percent are unwilling to make lifestyle changes.[64] Yet there are positive steps to be taken by healthcare workers. A study comparing those who noted internal barrier to change (lack of will power, too lazy) and external barriers (no transport, cost of joining a club) suggested that those who are aware of external limitations might be in a better position to circumvent them.[65] What can clinicians do in a busy office practice?[66]

- Ask about nutrition, exercise, and smoking habits as part of the vital signs.
- Ask if the patient is willing to change at this time[67] (simple questions regarding diet can identify a patient with greater than 30 percent of calories from total fat).
- Ask whether the barriers to change are internal or external.
- Offer assistance in helping the patient develop lifestyle habits. Point out that many are able to do this successfully, though not everyone succeeds at first.
- Arrange for a follow-up visit to monitor compliance and to mutually solve problems.
- Find out about and use health professionals such as registered dietitians, physiatrists, and exercise counselors.
- Finally – and perhaps most importantly – consider being a role model by

promoting a therapeutic diet with regular physical activity and avoiding excess calories that lead to overweight and obesity.

REFERENCES

1. Summary of the second report of the National Cholesterol Education Program (NCEP) expert panel on detection, evaluation, and treatment of high blood cholesterol in adults (Adult Treatment Panel II). *JAMA* 1993; **269**: 3015–23.
2. Appel LJ, Moore TJ, Obarzanek E, *et al*. A clinical trial of the effects of dietary patterns on blood pressure. *N Engl J Med* 1997; **336**: 1117–24.
3. Svetkey LP, Simons-Morton D, Vollmer WM, Appel LJ, Conlin PR, Ryan DH, Kennedy AJ. Effects of dietary patterns on blood pressure: subgroup analysis of the Dietary Approaches to Stop Hypertension (DASH) randomized clinical trial. *Arch Intern Med* 1999; **159**: 285–93.
4. Manson JE, Colditz GA, Stampfer MJ, *et al*. A prospective study of obesity and risk of coronary heart disease in women. *N Engl J Med* 1990; **322**: 882–9.
5. Hjermann I, Holme, I, Leren P. Oslo Study diet and anti smoking trial results after 102 months. *Am J Med* 1986; **80** (Suppl. 2A): 7–12.
6. Singh RB, Rastogi SS, Verma R, Laxmi B, Singh R, Ghosh S, Niaz MA. Randomized controlled trial of cardioprotective diet in patients with recent myocardial infarction: results of one year follow up. *Br Med J* 1992; **304**: 1015–19.
7. de Lorgeril M, Salen P, Martin JL, *et al*. Mediterranean diet, traditional risk factors, and the rate of cardiovascular complications after myocardial infarction: final report of the Lyon Diet Heart Study. *Circulation* 1999; **99**: 779–85.
8. Kris-Etherton P, Eckel RH, Howard BV, *et al*. Lyon Diet Heart Study. Benefits of a Mediterranean-style, National Cholesterol Education Program/American Heart Association Step I Dietary pattern on cardiovascular disease. *Circulation* 2001; **103**: 1823–5.
9. Schuler G, Hambrecht R, Schlierf G, *et al*. Regular physical exercise and low-fat diet effects of progression on coronary artery disease. *Circulation* 1992; **86**: 1–11.
10. Niebauer J, Hambrecht R, Velich, T, *et al*. Predictive value of lipid profile for salutary coronary angiographic changes in patients on a low-fat diet and physical exercise program. *Am J Cardiol* 1996; **78**: 163–7.
11. Watts GF, Lewis, B, Brunt JNH, Lewis ES, Coltart DJ, Smith LDR, Mann JI, Swan AV. Effects of coronary artery disease of lipid lowering diet, or diet plus cholestyramine in the St. Thomas Atherosclerosis Regression Study (STARS). *Lancet* 1992; **339**: 563–9.
12. Watts GF, Jackson P, Mandalia S, Brunt JN, Lewis ES, Coltart DJ, Lewis B. Nutrient intake and progression of coronary artery disease. *Am J Cardiol* 1994; **73**: 328–32.
13. Quinn TG, Alderman EL, McMillan A, Haskell W for the SCRIP investigators. Development of new coronary atherosclerotic lesions during a 4-year multifactor risk reduction program: The Stanford Risk Intervention Project (SCRIP). *J Am Coll Cardiol* 1994; **24**: 900–8.
14. Ornish D, Brown SE, Scherwitz LW, *et al*. Can lifestyle changes reverse coronary heart disease? The Lifestyle Heart Trial. *Lancet* 1990; **335**: 129–33.
15. Leaf A, Jorgensen MB, Jacobs AK, *et al*. Do fish oils prevent restenosis after coronary angioplasty? *Circulation* 1994; **90**: 2248–57.
16. Burr ML, Fehily AM, Gilbert JF, *et al*. Effects of changes in fat, fish, and fibre intakes on death and myocardial reinfarction: diet and reinfarction trial (DART). *Lancet* 1989; **2**: 757–61.

17. Siscovick DS, Raghunathan TE, King I, *et al.* Dietary intake and cell membrane levels of long-chain n-3 polyunsaturated fatty acids and the risk of primary cardiac arrest. *JAMA* 1995; **274**: 1363–7.
18. de Lorgeril M, Renaud S, Marnelle N, *et al.* Mediterranean alpha-linolenic acid rich diet in secondary prevention of coronary heart disease. *Lancet* 1994; **343**: 1454–9.
19. Cobb MM, Teitelbaum HS, Breslow JL. Lovastatin efficacy in reducing low-density lipoprotein cholesterol levels on high- vs low-fat diets. *JAMA* 1991; **265**: 997–1001.
20. Hunninghake DB, Stein EA, Dujovne CA, *et al.* The efficacy of intensive dietary therapy alone or combined with lovastatin in outpatients with hypercholesterolemia. *N Engl J Med* 1993; **328**: 12131–9.
21. Yusuf, S, Anand S. Cost of prevention. The case of lipid lowering. *Circulation* 1996; **93**: 1774–6.
22. Krauss RM, Eckel RH, Howard B, *et al.* AHA Dietary Guidelines: revision 2000: a statement for healthcare professionals from the Nutrition Committee of the American Heart Association. *Circulation* 2000; **102**: 2284–99.
23. Executive Summary of the Third Report of the National Cholesterol Education Program (NCEP) Expert Panel on Detection, Evaluation, and Treatment of High Blood Cholesterol in Adults (Adult Treatment Panel III). *JAMA* 2001; **285**: 2486–97.
24. Keys A, *et al.* Seven Countries – *A Multivariate Analysis of Death and Coronary Heart Disease. A Commonwealth Fund Book.* Cambridge, Massachusetts: Harvard University Press; 1980; 1–381.
25. Ginsberg HN, Kris-Etherton P, Dennis B, *et al.* Effects of reducing dietary saturated fatty acids on plasma lipids and lipoproteins in healthy subjects: the DELTA study, protocol 1. *Arterioscler Thromb Vasc Biol* 1998; **18**: 441–9.
26. Barr SL, Ramakrishnan R, Johnson C, Holleran S, Dell RB, Ginsberg HN. Reducing total dietary fat without reducing saturated fatty acids does not significantly lower total plasma cholesterol concentrations in normal males. *Am J Clin Nutr* 1992; **55**: 675–81.
27. Ascherio A, Rimm EB, Giovannucci EL, Spiegelman D, Stampfer M, Willett WC. Dietary fat and risk of coronary heart disease in men: cohort follow up study in the United States. *Br Med J* 1996; **313**: 84–90.
28. Watts GF, Lewis B, Jackson P, Burke V, Lewis ES, Brunt JN, Coltart DJ. Relationships between nutrient intake and progression/regression of coronary atherosclerosis as assessed by serial quantitative angiography. *Can J Cardiol* 1995; **11** (Suppl. G): 110G–114G.
29. Stamler J, Shekelle R. Dietary cholesterol and human coronary heart disease. *Arch Pathol Lab Med* 1988; **112**: 1032–40.
30. Shekelle RB, Shyrcck AM, Paul O, *et al.* Diet, serum cholesterol, and death from coronary heart disease: The Western Electric Study. *N Engl J Med* 1981: **304**; 65–70.
31. Lichtenstein AH, Kennedy E, Barrier P, *et al.* Dietary fat consumption and health. *Nutr Rev* 1998; **56** (5 Pt 2): S3–19.
32. Connor WE, Connor SL. Should a low-fat, high carbohydrate diet be recommended for everyone? *N Engl J Med* 1997; **337**: 562–3; discussion 566–7.
33. Katan MB, Grundy SM, Willett WC. Beyond low fat diets. *N Engl J Med* 1997; **337**: 563–6; discussion 566–7.
34. Leaf A. Editorial. Dietary prevention of coronary heart disease. The Lyon Diet Heart Study. *Circulation* 1999; **99**: 733–5.
35. Meydani SN, Lichtenstein AH, Cornwall S, *et al.* Immunologic effects of a National Cholesterol Education Panel. Step-2. Diets with and without fish-derived n-3 fatty acid enrichment. *J Clin Invest* 1993; **92**: 105–13.

36. Rissanen T, Voutilainen S, Nyyssonen K, Lakka TA, Salonen JT. Fish oil-derived fatty acids, docosahexaenoic acid and docosapentaenoic acid, and the risk of acute coronary events. The Kuopio Ischaemic Heart Disease Risk Factor Study. *Circulation* 2000; **102**: 2677.

37. Lichtenstein AH, Van Horn L. Very low fat diets. AHA Science Advisory *Circulation* 1998; **98**: 935–9.

38. Marckmann P, Gronbaek M. Fish consumption and coronary heart disease mortality. A systematic review of prospective cohort studies. *Eur J Clin Nutr* 1999; **53**: 585–90.

39. GISSI-Prevenzione Investigators (Gruppo Italiano per lo Studio della Sopravvivenza nell'Infarto miocardico). Dietary supplementation with n-3 polyunsaturated fatty acids and vitamin E after myocardial infarction: results of the GISSI-Prevenzione trial. *Lancet* 1999; **354**: 447–55.

40. Van Horn L. Fiber, lipids, and coronary heart disease: a statement for healthcare professionals from the Nutrition Committee, American Heart Association For the Nutrition Committee. *Circulation* 1997; **95**: 2701–4.

41. Miettinen TA, Puska, P, Gylling H, Vanhanen H, Vartiarien E. Reduction of serum cholesterol with sitostanol-ester margarine in a mildly hypercholesterolemic population. *N Engl J Med* 1995; **333**: 1308–12.

42. Pearson TA. Alcohol and heart disease. *Circulation* 1996; **94**: 3023–5.

43. Rimm EB, Williams P, Fosher, Criqui, M, Stampfer MJ. Moderate alcohol intake and lower risk of coronary heart disease: meta-analysis of effects on lipids and haemostatic factors. *Br Med J* 1999; **319**: 1523–8.

44. Rimm EB, Klatsky A, Grobbee D, Stampfer MJ. Review of moderate alcohol consumption and reduced risk of coronary heart disease: is the effect due to beer, wine, or spirits. *Br Med J* 1996; **312**: 731–6.

45. Law M, Wald N. Why heart disease mortality is low in France: the time lag explanation. *Br Med J* 1999; **318**: 1471–80.

46. Frost G, Leeds AA, Doré CJ, Madeiros S, Brading S, Dornhorst A. Glycaemic index as a determinant of serum HDL-cholesterol concentration *Lancet* 1999; **353**: 1269–76.

47. Wood PD, Stefanick ML, Williams PT, Haskell WL. The effects on plasma lipoproteins of a prudent weight-reducing diet with or without exercise, in overweight men and women. *N Engl J Med* 1991; **325**: 461–6.

48. Huttunen JK, Lansimies E, Voutilainen E, *et al*. Effect of moderate physical exercise in serum lipoproteins: a controlled clinical trial with special reference to serum high density lipoproteins. *Circulation* 1979; **6**: 1220–9.

49. Tribble DL. Antioxidant consumption and risk of coronary heart disease: emphasis on vitamin C, vitamin E and B carotene. *Circulation* 1999; **99**: 591–5.

50. Kushi LH, Folsom AR, Prineas RJ, Mink PJ, Wu Y, Bostick RM. Dietary antioxidant vitamins and death from coronary heart disease in postmenopausal women. *N Engl J Med* 1996; **334**: 1156–62.

51. Hu FB, Stampfer MJ, Manson JE, *et al*. Frequent nut consumption and risk of coronary heart disease in women: prospective cohort study. *Br Med J* 1998; **317**: 1341–5.

52. Stephans NG, Parsons A, Schofield PM, Kelly F, Cheeseman K, Mitchinson MJ, Brown MJ. Randomized controlled trial of vitamin E in patients with coronary disease: Cambridge Heart Antioxidant Study (CHAOS). *Lancet* 1996; **347**: 781–6.

53. Yusuf S, Dagenais G, Pogue J, Bosch J, Sleight P. Vitamin E supplementation and cardiovascular events in high-risk patients. The Heart Outcomes Prevention Evaluation Study Investigators. *N Engl J Med* 2000; **342**: 154–60.

54. Heart Protection Study, presented at annual meetings of American Heart Association, Anaheim, California, November 2001.

55. Brown BG, Zhao X-Q, Chait A, *et al.* Simvastatin and niacin, antioxidant vitamins, or the combination for the prevention of coronary disease. *N Engl J Med* 2001; **345**: 1583–92.

56. Hennekens CH, Buring JE, Manson JE, *et al.* Lack of effect of long-term supplementation with beta carotene on the incidence of malignant neoplasms and cardiovascular disease. *N Engl J Med* 1996; **334**: 1145–9.

57. Omenn GS, Goodman GE, Thornquist MD, *et al.* Effects of a combination of beta carotene and vitamin A on lung cancer and cardiovascular disease. *N Engl J Med* 1996; **334**: 1150–5.

58. α-Tocopherol, β-Carotene Prevention Study Group. The effect of vitamin E and beta carotene on the incidence of lung cancer and other cancers in male smokers. *N Engl J Med* 1994; **330**: 1029–35.

59. Malinow MR, Bostom AG, Krauss RM. Homocyst(e)ine, diet, and cardiovascular diseases. AHA Science Advisory. *Circulation* 1999; **99**: 178–82.

60. Selhub J, Jacques PF, Wilson PWF, Rush D, Rosenberg IH. Vitamin status and intake as primary determinants of homocysteinemia in an elderly population. *JAMA* 1993; **270**: 2693–8.

61. Rimm EB, Willett WC, Hu FB, *et al.* Folate and vitamin B6 from diet and supplements in relation to risk of coronary heart disease among women. *JAMA* 1998; **278**; 359–64.

62. Schnyder G, Roffi M, Pin R, *et al.* Decreased rate of coronary stenosis after lowering of plasma homocysteine levels. *N Engl J Med* 2001; **345**: 1593–2000.

63. Tuomilehto J, Lindstrom J, Eriksson JG, *et al.* Prevention of Type 2 diabetes mellitus by changes in lifestyle among subjects with impaired glucose tolerance. *N Engl J Med* 2001; **344**; 1343–50.

64. Cheney CD. Medical nonadherence: a behavioral analysis. In: Cautela J, Ishaq W (eds). *Contemporary Issues in Behavior Therapy: Improving the Human Condition.* New York: Plenum Press, 1996: 9–21.

65. Ziebland S, Thorogood M, Yudkin P, Jones L, Coulter A. Lack of willpower or lack of wherewithal? 'Internal' and 'external' barriers to changing diet and exercise in a three year follow-up of participants in a health check. *Soc Sci Med* 1998; **46**: 461–5.

66. Sherman SE. Commentary. *ACP Journal Club*, 1999; page 16.

67. Greene GW, Rossi SR, Reed GR, Willey C, Prochaska JO. Stages of change for reducing dietary fat to 30 percent of energy or less. *J Am Diet Assoc* 1994; **94**: 1105–10; quiz 1111–12.

8

Drug treatment of dyslipoproteinemia

DONALD B HUNNINGHAKE

INTRODUCTION

Atherosclerosis involving the coronary, carotid, and peripheral vasculature is the leading cause of death, both in the United States and in many other parts of the world. There are many risk factors for the development of cardiovascular disease, but lipid and lipoprotein abnormalities play a major role. It has now been established conclusively in controlled clinical trials that reducing the levels of total and low-density lipoprotein (LDL)-cholesterol reduces the risk of coronary heart disease (CHD) in both primary and secondary prevention in men and women, and up to the age of 75 years (see Chapter 1). Clinical events are also reduced in the carotid and peripheral vasculature and in diabetes mellitus with low-density lipoprotein-cholesterol (LDL-C) lowering. High-density lipoprotein (HDL)-cholesterol levels have been shown in epidemiological studies to be inversely related to CHD risk, and there is fairly strong evidence from clinical trials that HDL-cholesterol (HDL-C) raising reduces CHD risk, though the proof of this suggestion is not conclusive. Epidemiological studies have also shown elevated triglyceride levels to be an independent risk factor for developing CHD. Moreover, there is a strong suggestion that other triglyceride-rich particles, including intermediate-density lipoprotein (IDL), very low-density lipoprotein (VLDL) remnants and the associated smaller, more dense LDL particles are also important predictors of risk. However, there is as yet not conclusive evidence from large clinical trials that the lowering of triglycerides and associated lipoprotein abnormalities is associated with reduced risk in those patients who have achieved target LDL-C levels.

Based upon the evidence discussed in greater depth in previous chapters, the National Cholesterol Education Program (NCEP) has established LDL-C as the primary target for therapy. In patients with low HDL-C, LDL-C lowering is recommended, but therapies which also increase HDL-C levels are likewise recommended. Reducing triglyceride levels and all the associated atherogenic lipoprotein abnormalities in this group is recommended in high-risk individuals such as those with CHD or in whom other risk factors are present. In patients with very high triglyceride levels, triglyceride lowering is also recommended in order to reduce the risk for pancreatitis.

MAJOR CLASSES OF DRUGS

The major classes of lipid-lowering drugs include:

- Hexamethylglutaryl-coenzyme A (HMG-CoA) reductase inhibitors (statins)
- Bile-acid sequestrants (resins)
- Nicotinic acid or niacin
- Fibric acid derivatives (fibrates)

The statins are used primarily for lowering LDL-C, but they also produce moderate reductions in triglycerides in hypertriglyceridemic patients and modest increases in HDL-C levels. The resins are used exclusively for lowering LDL-C. Nicotinic acid favorably affects all lipoproteins that are associated with increased risk for CHD, and this is the most effective class for increasing HDL-C levels and produces significant reductions in triglycerides and moderate decreases in LDL-C. The fibrates are used primarily for triglyceride lowering, and can produce significant increases in HDL-C, especially in hypertriglyceridemic patients. The effects on LDL-C are usually minimal, but significant increases in LDL-C levels may be seen in hyper-triglyceridemic patients. A summary of the effects of the four classes of drugs on lipid and lipoprotein levels is presented in Table 8.1.

Table 8.1 *Summary of the effect of the various classes of drugs on lipid and lipoprotein levels*

	Decreased LDL-C (%)	Increased HDL-C (%)	Decreased triglyceride (%)
Statins	18–60	5–15[a]	7–30[b]
Resins	15–30	3–5	No effect or increase
Nicotinic acid	5–25	15–40	20–50[b]
Fibrates	5–20[c,d]	10–25[a]	20–70[b]

[a]Greatest increase if baseline HDL-cholesterol (HDL-C) is low or if hypertriglyceridemia is present.
[b]Greatest decreases usually observed in more severe forms of hypertriglyceridemia.
[c]Differences among drug in class.
[d]Increased in hypertriglyceridemia.

STATINS

The statins are currently the most widely prescribed class of drugs, and are the most effective class for lowering LDL-C levels – the primary target for treatment in the NCEP guidelines. In prospective and retrospective analyses of clinical trials, the statins have been shown to reduce essentially every clinical manifestation of the atherosclerotic process in all arterial beds. Benefit has been demonstrated in both men and women, and in primary and secondary prevention (see Chapter 1). The statins have been documented as being safe in long-term clinical trials, they are easy to administer, are associated with few drug–drug interactions, and both their patient and physician acceptance is generally good.

There are currently five statin drugs that have been approved for clinical use in the United States:

- Lovastatin (Mevacor®)
- Pravastatin (Pravachol®)
- Simvastatin (Zocor®)
- Fluvastatin (Lescol®)
- Atorvastatin (Lipitor®)

Lipid and lipoprotein effects

With the currently approved doses of the statins, reductions in LDL-C of 18–60 percent have been reported.[1] These reductions in LDL-C are dose-dependent, but log-linear; thus, for every doubling of the statin dose after the starting dose, an additional 6 percent decrease in LDL-C levels is noted. In patients with hyper-triglyceridemia, the percentage reductions in LDL-C levels per milligram of drug administered tends to be less than in non-hypertriglyceridemic patients. There are rare patients who cannot achieve a 15 percent reduction in LDL-C levels with statin therapy, and the mechanisms for this reduced response have not been clearly defined. Some of these patients may be true non-responders, but some may also be non-compliers. Some other causes of poor response may include secondary causes of hyperlipoproteinemia such as untreated or inadequately treated hypothyroidism.

The reported decrease in reduction in triglyceride levels is generally between 7 and 30 percent. In patients with triglyceride levels of less than 150–200 mg/dL, there is no consistent or dose–response effect on triglyceride levels. In individuals with triglyceride levels of >200–250 mg/dL, the percentage lowering of triglycerides closely resembles the percentage lowering of LDL-C.

The increases in HDL-C levels in clinical trials has been in the range of 5–15 percent, but there is no clear-cut dose–response effect. The increase in HDL-C levels is generally greater in patients with either low HDL-C and/or elevated triglycerides at baseline. In several clinical trials, the greatest percentage reduction – as well as absolute reduction in risk – occurred with statin-induced reductions in LDL-C, even though there was little or no effect on HDL-C levels.[2]

Mechanism of action

Statins inhibit HMG-CoA reductase, the rate-limiting step in cholesterol bio-synthesis. Hepatocyte cholesterol content is decreased, resulting in an increased population of LDL receptors and reduced serum LDL levels. IDL and VLDL remnants are also removed by the LDL receptor; this mechanism might partially account for the decreased levels of triglycerides and triglyceride-rich lipoproteins. In some patients, the hepatic release or synthesis of lipoproteins is also decreased with statins. The decreased release of lipoproteins (VLDL) may also account for some of the decrease in triglycerides and triglyceride-rich particles. Although the effect is modest, this mechanism may also account for the lowering of LDL-C levels in LDL-receptor-negative patients with homozygous hypercholesterolemia. The statins also reduce the concentration of all LDL particles, including the smaller, more dense particles. Depending upon the degree of triglyceride lowering, they may not alter LDL composition, but the reduction in the number of smaller, more dense LDL particles is dose-dependent and tends to be greater than that obtained with either niacin or fibrates. There is currently considerable interest in whether statins reduce CHD risk by non-lipid mechanisms – usually referred to as pleotrophic effects. At present, clinically significant differences in pleotrophic effects among the statins has not been well established, and it is not known whether CHD risk reduction occurs beyond the effects of statins as inhibitors of cholesterol, mevalonate, or other intermediary products of cholesterol biosynthesis and their effects on triglycerides and triglyceride-rich particles. However, evidence is emerging of other effects such as increased bone density and decreased fracture rates.[3]

Side effects

A wide variety of adverse effects of statins has infrequently been associated with statin administration, including rash, allergic reactions, and gastrointestinal complaints. However, the areas that have generated the greatest interest clinically have been elevations of transaminase levels and muscle pains or myopathy.

TRANSAMINASE ELEVATIONS

All lipid-lowering drugs have a tendency to increase serum transaminase levels shortly after initiation of therapy, but the values then generally return to baseline. Discussion and disagreement persist, however, as to whether elevated transaminase levels represent hepatotoxicity and whether chronic administration of drug in a patient with elevated transaminase levels would lead to chronic liver disease. There are occasional reports of a hepatitis-like picture associated with statin administration with elevated transaminase levels and an influenza-like syndrome with fatigue and anorexia. Most of the increases in transaminase associated with statins occur during the first few months after drug therapy is initiated. Although there may be some disagreement regarding the clinical significance of elevated transaminase levels, the usual and prudent approach is to reduce the dose of drug or discontinue if transaminase elevations are persistently more than three-fold upper limit of normal (ULN). The incidence is dose-dependent, but generally ranges from 0.5 to 2 percent for the various statins. If elevations persist, the statin should be discontinued. If persistent increases in the range of two- to three-fold ULN are noted, then the statin dose is usually reduced. Other causes of transaminase elevations such as concomitant drug therapy, alcohol, or other hepatotoxins must always be considered.

When the transaminase levels return to normal, re-challenge with a statin should be considered if major reductions in LDL-C levels are required to achieve target goal. The initial dose should be less than the dose that the patient was receiving when the transaminase elevation occurred. Some patients will tolerate the same statin when re-challenged, but arbitrary selection of another statin for re-challenge should also be considered. The transaminase levels should be monitored more carefully following the initial re-challenge. A single episode of transaminase elevation should not be considered a reason to never consider statin therapy again. The suggested frequency of monitoring of transaminase levels by the Food and Drug Administration has been decreasing (see Physicians' Desk Reference for individual statins). However, many patients have an inordinate fear of statin-induced hepatotoxicity, and routine monitoring at each clinic visit may be necessary in some patients in order to maintain compliance.

MUSCLE PAINS AND MYOPATHY

There are probably three broad categories in this area, though the terminology employed in the literature has not been consistent. However, the clinical significance of each of the three groups is quite different.

- Myalgia: this term is used to indicate muscle complaints without an elevation of creatine kinase (CK) levels. Myalgia or non-specific joint pains are probably the most common complaint causing discontinuance of statin therapy. The muscle and joint pains disappear when statin therapy is discontinued, and reappear when statin therapy is re-initiated. In placebo-controlled clinical trials, the incidence of these complaints is essentially the same in the placebo and statin-treated groups. There is no evidence that patients with these chronic complaints progress to more severe forms of myopathy, or that any muscle damage is occurring, or that rhabdomyolysis will occur. CK measurements should be carried out and, if normal, the patient should be informed that there is no evidence of muscle damage. Isolated CK elevations of less than three-fold ULN should not be considered clinically significant. Most of the complaints in this group of patients are probably not truly statin-related. The arbitrary switching from one statin to another may occasionally be successful.
- Myositis: these patients have increased CK levels, but without muscle symptoms. Asymptomatic increases in CK values are quite common, even in patients who are not receiving statin therapy. The most common cause is exercise during the period before the blood test is performed, or a marked increase in exercise. In clinical trials, an asymptomatic increase in CK level to >10-fold ULN, confirmed by a repeat measurement, has been used as the criterion for discontinuing statin therapy. Generally, repeat measurements of CK levels are carried out if the CK values are more than three-fold ULN. The cautious approach would be initially to reduce the statin dose if the CK value persistently remains above three-fold ULN and no other cause can be found. If CK elevations more than three-fold

ULN persist, the original statin drug can be discontinued, but re-challenge with another statin drug should be considered if major reductions in LDL-C are required to achieve target levels. There is no good evidence that asymptomatic modest increases in CK levels progress to more severe forms of myopathy, including rhabdomyolysis. Routine monitoring of CK levels is not recommended as they do not predict the development of more severe forms of myopathy, and simply cause confusion.

- Myopathy: these patients have muscle pains with elevated CK levels. They are the patients who can progress to rhabdomyolysis and potential renal failure if drug is not discontinued promptly. Patients with this type of myopathy have CK levels that are usually considerably greater than 10-fold ULN. Routine monitoring of CK does not predict development of myopathy. It is extremely important to instruct patients to report promptly any generalized muscle aching, weakness, and 'flu-like' symptoms. Adequate instruction of patients is the most important preventive measure for avoiding severe complications. Myopathy rarely occurs with the higher statin doses, but is frequently associated with the co-administration of other drugs which decrease the hepatic metabolism of statins and higher blood levels. With the exception of pravastatin, the statins are metabolized by the cytochrome P-450 system.[4] Many non-statin drugs utilize the 3A4 type of cytochrome P-450, as do atorvastatin, simvastatin, and lovastatin, whereas fluvastatin utilizes the 2C9 type. Drugs involving an interaction with 3A4 may be associated with myopathy. The most common drugs associated with statin myopathy include erythromycin and other macrolide antibiotics, antifungal agents, protease inhibitors, and cyclosporine. Fibrates can occasionally cause myopathy when administered as monotherapy, but have frequently been reported to do so when co-administered with statins. Gemfibrozil has been implicated more frequently than fenofibrate in this respect. The older sustained-release preparations of nicotinic acid may initially cause hepatotoxicity, followed by myopathy if co-administered with a statin. Other nicotinic acid preparations have rarely been associated with myopathy.

Effect on CHD risk

Statin utilization in clinical trials has been associated with reductions in total mortality, myocardial infarction (MI), revascularization procedures, and stroke (see Chapter 1). One meta-analysis of 30 817 participants indicated that a 28 percent reduction in LDL-C over a mean treatment period of 5.4 years was associated with a 21 percent decrease in all-cause mortality and a 31 percent decrease in major coronary events.[5] These effects were noted in men and women up to the age of 75 years in both primary and secondary prevention trials. The Heart Protection Study[6] reported benefit up to the age of 80 years at entry into the study. Additionally, benefit has been demonstrated in both the native coronary arteries and vein grafts and in patients with diabetes mellitus.[7,8] Retrospective analyses have shown reductions in essentially all clinical events related to atherosclerosis in all arterial beds.

Major clinical uses

The statins can be used in any patient where LDL-C lowering is required to achieve target LDL-C levels. They are also very useful in patients with combined hyperlipidemia (both elevated cholesterol and triglycerides) because of their additional significant triglyceride-lowering effects. The statins lower the concentration of all the LDL particles (both the smaller, more dense as well as the larger, more buoyant) as well as IDL and VLDL remnants. In patients with low HDL-C levels and high LDL-C, aggressive lowering of LDL-C attenuates much of the risk associated with low HDL-C levels. In fact, these patients achieve greater benefit from the lowering of LDL-C levels. It is difficult to define an exact algorithm for use in patients who primarily have hypertriglyceridemia. If triglyceride elevations are the major abnormality, then other drugs should be considered. Non-statin drugs are almost always preferred for initial therapy in patients with triglyceride levels >750 mg/dL. Patients with triglyceride levels >1000 mg/dL are especially prone to develop pancreatitis, and other therapies (e.g. fibrates and omega-3 fatty acids) should be considered initially.

RESINS

The resins are used primarily for lowering LDL-C levels in patients without significant hypertriglyceridemia. They were the first class of drugs to demonstrate that LDL-C lowering was conclusively associated with a reduction in CHD risk. Resins generally produce modest reductions in LDL-C, in the range of 15–25 percent. They can be used in combination with statins, nicotinic acid and fibrates for additional control of lipid and lipoprotein abnormalities. The major advantages are that they do reduce CHD risk, are non-absorbable drugs, and have no significant long-term toxicity. The major disadvantages are that the granular forms of these drugs are difficult to administer, the frequency of both upper and lower gastrointestinal complaints is high, and acceptance by both patients and health professionals is low. The available drugs in this class include:

- Cholestyramine (Questran®)
- Cholestyramine granules (Questran-Light®)
- Colestipol granules (Colestid®)
- Colestipol tablets (Colestid®)
- Colesevelam tablets (WelChol®)

Lipid and lipoprotein effects

The primary effect of this class of drug is to reduce LDL-C levels, with usual reductions in the range of 15–25 percent being reported, though 30 percent reductions have been reported with either 24 g of cholestyramine or 30 g of colestipol. Mean reductions in LDL-C of 12–18 percent have been observed with the recently approved colesevelam when administered in a total daily dose of 2.5–3.8 g.[9]

The resins produce modest increases in HDL-C, in the range of 3–5 percent. The resins usually have no effect on triglyceride levels when pretreatment values are <200 mg/dL. However, if triglyceride levels are >200 mg/dL, then modest increases may be expected, with major increases if the levels are >400 mg/dL. This is usually considered as an absolute contra-indication to resins as monotherapy. In addition, when resins are used as monotherapy in patients with the rare genetic disorder, dysbetalipoproteinemia or Type III hyperlipoproteinemia, major increases in cholesterol and triglycerides are observed.

Mechanism of action

The resins bind bile acids in the intestine through anion exchange; the resin–bile acid complex thus formed is not absorbed from the intestine. This reduces the enterohepatic recirculation of bile acids, increases fecal bile acid excretion, and enhances the conversion of cholesterol to bile acids in the liver. The decrease in hepatocyte cholesterol content increases LDL receptor expression and a lowering of serum LDL-C levels. The resins may also increase HMG-CoA reductase activity and hepatic VLDL production, and increase serum triglyceride levels. Co-administration of a statin prevents the increase in HMG-CoA reductase activity. Resin plus statin is an effective combination for LDL-C lowering as the two drugs enhance LDL receptor expression, albeit by different mechanisms.

Side effects

Resin therapy may produce a variety of upper and lower gastrointestinal symptoms, including bloating, fullness, nausea, abdominal pain, flatulence, and constipation. It is usually best to start with one or two unit doses of resins per day and to test various vehicles. Changing the vehicle may decrease some objections to the taste and the sandy, gritty consistency of the granules of cholestyramine and colestipol. When the best regimen for administration has been determined, the dose may be increased. The resins may also bind other drugs that are co-administered and hence decrease their absorption. Although the absorption of many drugs is not decreased with resins, the general recommendation is that other drugs should be taken either 1 h before or 4 h after the administration of a resin. As many patients take most of their other medications in the morning, the resin is best administered in the evening. Preliminary evidence with colesevelam, which is administered in tablet form, suggests fewer gastrointestinal complaints and less effect on drug absorption than occur with the older resins. Unfortunately, colesevelam administration requires the patient to take four to six large tablets each day.

CHD risk

The resins were used in the Lipid Research Clinics Coronary Primary Prevention Study, which was the first large clinical trial to demonstrate conclusively that LDL-C reduction decreased the incidence of fatal and non-fatal MI.[10] A less well-controlled trial with colestipol demonstrated a decrease in total mortality. Several angiographic trials have also demonstrated decreased rates of progression when resins were used either as monotherapy (STARS, NHLBI type II study) or in combination therapy (FATS, CLAS). Ileal bypass surgery, which works by a mechanism similar to resin therapy but is more effective in increasing fecal bile-acid excretion, also dramatically reduces CHD risk.

Major uses

Currently, the resins are used primarily in patients without significant hyper-triglyceridemia who have not achieved their target LDL-C goals with statin therapy. The usual daily doses range from 4 to 16 g of cholestyramine, from 5 to 20 g of colestipol, and from 2.5 to 3.8 g of colesevelam. As they are non-absorbable drugs with no long-term toxicity, the resins are also used in women of childbearing potential, in children, and also in the occasional patient who does not want to take a systemic drug. Resins can be used in any patient where only modest LDL-C lowering is required, and they can also be used in combination with nicotinic acid and fibrates to provide lipid control in patients with multiple lipoprotein disorders.

NICOTINIC ACID

Nicotinic acid or niacin has a favorable effect on all the lipids and lipoproteins which affect CHD risk. Nicotinamide – which is sometimes confused with nicotinic acid – has only vitamin functions, and no lipid-altering effects. Nicotinic acid is the most effective drug for increasing HDL-C levels, and is also very effective in lowering triglyceride levels. The LDL-C lowering effects are usually modest. Limited data exist which indicate that nicotinic acid reduces the risk for CHD. The advantages of nicotinic acid are its favorable effects on all lipids and lipoproteins, including lipoprotein (a) [Lp(a)]. Many preparations are available as over-the-counter products, and these are relatively inexpensive. The disadvantage is that the side effects – especially vasodilatory effects of severe flushing – severely limit the use of niacin. The drug is not well accepted by patients, and considerable effort by both physicians and nursing staff is required to maintain compliance.

The available drugs in this class include:

- Crystalline nicotinic acid (multiple preparations)
- Sustained-release nicotinic acid (multiple preparations)
- Niaspan®
- Advicor® (combination of Niaspan® and Mevacor®)

Lipid and lipoprotein effects

Nicotinic acid is the most effective drug for increasing HDL-C levels. Although increases of as much as 40 percent have been reported, the usual increase is in the range of 15–30 percent. Small doses, which may be tolerated (e.g. 750–1000 mg), may increase HDL-C by 15 percent, have a minimal effect on triglyceride levels, and have no effect on LDL-C levels. The older sustained-release preparations are not as effective for increasing HDL-C as crystalline nicotinic acid or Niaspan. The reported effect of nicotinic acid on LDL-C lowering in controlled studies varies considerably, and may be somewhat greater in patients with associated hypertriglyceridemia. Generally, reductions in LDL-C of 10–15 percent are observed with doses of 1.5 g/day, and 15–25 percent with doses of 3.0–4.5 g/day, though these higher doses are rarely tolerated. Nicotinic acid also lowers triglyceride levels by 20–50 percent. The greater reductions are usually with high doses of nicotinic acid in more severe hypertriglyceridemic patients. Nicotinic acid lowers the concentration of triglycerides, VLDL, IDL and triglyceride-rich lipoprotein particles which are believed to be atherogenic. It also causes a shift in the composition of LDL particles from the small dense particles (more atherogenic) to the larger, buoyant particles. There is a modest decrease in the total number of LDL particles. Usually, there is no increase in serum LDL-C levels when nicotinic acid is administered in hyper-triglyceridemic patients. Although the clinical significance in terms of CHD risk reduction has not been established, nicotinic acid and estrogen are the only drugs that lower Lp(a) levels. The decreases in Lp(a) appear to be dose-dependent, and reductions of up to 30 percent have been noted with the higher doses of nicotinic acid.

Mechanism of action

Nicotinic acid appears to alter lipid levels by inhibiting the synthesis of lipoproteins and decreasing the synthesis or release of lipoprotein particles by the liver. Since VLDL is the precursor of VLDL remnants, IDL and LDL, the concentration of all of these lipoproteins is reduced. Nicotinic acid also increases apolipoprotein A and HDL levels.

Effect on CHD risk

Very limited data exist on the ability of nicotinic acid to reduce the risk of CHD. A reduction in fatal and non-fatal MI was reported in the Coronary Drug Project, and the long-term follow-up of this study showed a reduction in mortality.[11] Nicotinic acid has also been shown to reduce the rates of progression in three angiographic trials when combined with resin or statin therapy. Likewise, a reduction in mortality was also reported when nicotinic acid was combined with clofibrate in the Stockholm Ischemic Heart Disease study.

Major uses

Nicotinic acid is used primarily in the treatment of atherogenic dyslipidemia characterized by low HDL-C and elevated triglyceride levels. The usual daily doses of crystalline nicotinic acid range from 1 to 3 g per day, or from 1 to 2 g per day for the sustained-release preparations and Niaspan. However, many of these patients may have diabetes mellitus or insulin resistance. Nicotinic acid, especially at the higher doses, may make the control of diabetes more difficult. Recent data obtained with the use of Niaspan suggest that this compound can be safely administered to most diabetics, albeit with care. The diagnosis of insulin resistance is more difficult to establish on routine clinical evaluation; central obesity and hypertension are clues. The fibrates are generally preferred over nicotinic acid in this situation. Nicotinic acid is definitely the most effective drug for increasing HDL-C levels and is very effective, even in patients who do not have hypertriglyceridemia. It can also be used as monotherapy for lowering LDL-C levels, though the required dose is usually high and significant side effects frequently result. There may be a cost benefit with nicotinic acid if the patient is able to tolerate it. Currently, nicotinic acid is used most frequently in combination with statins for the management of combined hyper-lipidemia; it can also be used together with resins, but this combination leads to a higher incidence of side effects. Niacin can also be used in combination with fibrates, primarily for management of hypertriglyceridemia.

FIBRATES

The fibrates are primarily used for lowering triglyceride levels. They produce modest increases in HDL-C levels and modest decreases in LDL-C levels, though in hypertriglyceridemic patients they can significantly increase LDL-C levels. The fibrates alter the composition of LDL by increasing cholesterol ester and decreasing triglyceride content. The fibrates decrease the concentration of small, dense LDL particles, increase the concentration of large buoyant LDL particles, and may modestly decrease the total number of LDL particles. They have been shown to reduce the risk of fatal and non-fatal MI and stroke, though a decrease in total mortality has not been documented. Earlier studies suggested an increase in non-CHD mortality, but recent studies have not confirmed this finding. The side effects are primarily gastrointestinal in nature, and they may increase the risk for gallstone formation.

The available preparations which are used in the United States include:

* Gemfibrozil (Lopid®)
* Fenofibrate (Tri-Cor®)

Side effects

The fibrates are generally well tolerated in most patients, with gastrointestinal complaints – both upper and lower – being the most common side effect. Abdominal discomfort, heartburn, flatulence, and diarrhea are some of the more common complaints. The fibrates increase the lithogenicity of bile, and consequently the risk for gallstone formation is increased. Fibrates bind strongly to serum albumin, and drug interactions related to altered protein binding and increased free drug concentrations can occur; an increased anticoagulant effect of warfarin is a classic example of this. The fibrates are primarily excreted by the kidney, and so elevated levels may occur with decreased renal function. Myopathy has been observed in patients with reduced renal function or low serum albumin levels. Myopathy – and rarely also rhabdomyolysis – may occur when fibrates are administered in combination with statins.

Mechanism of action

The mechanism of action of the fibrates is not completely understood, and it may vary among the different members of the group. All fibrates increase lipoprotein lipase, which in turn increases the removal of fatty acids from triglyceride-rich particles. These smaller particles are more effectively removed by the LDL receptor. The fibrates may also increase fatty acid oxidation and decrease the formation of VLDL triglycerides. All of these actions result in a lowering of serum triglycerides. The smaller, more dense LDL particles are also transformed into larger, more buoyant LDL particles. Fibrates are also agonists for the nuclear transcription factor, peroxisome proliferation activation factor (PPAR). This mechanism may control many of the lipid-altering effects, as well as other atherogenic mechanisms.

Effect on CHD risk

A number of early small trials were conducted, the results of which indicated that clofibrate reduced CHD events. The World Health Organization (WHO) clofibrate study was a large trial in which it was demonstrated that clofibrate reduced coronary events, though there appeared to be an increase in non-CHD mortality and clofibrate has been very little used since then. The Helsinki Heart Study then demonstrated a reduction in fatal and non-fatal MI with gemfibrozil.[12] Subsequently, the prevention of angiographic progression in both native arteries and vein grafts was shown in men with low HDL levels. A recently completed trial of considerable interest is the Veteran's Administration Affairs High-Density Lipoprotein Cholesterol Intervention Trial (VA-HIT).[13] The results of this study showed that gemfibrozil reduced the risk of non-fatal MI, CHD death and stroke in men with low HDL-C levels, modest increases in triglycerides and low LDL-C levels. However, another study – the Bezafibrate Infarct Prevention (BIP) Study – did not show any significant reduction in CHD events in men with low HDL-C levels. Thus, confusion persists regarding the benefits of fibrates for reducing CHD risk. The totality of data indicates that fibrates do reduce the risk of non-fatal MI, CHD death, and stroke, but that total mortality has not been decreased.

Major clinical uses

Gemfibrozil is generally administered in a dosage of 600 mg twice daily, and fenofibrate as a single daily dose of 160 mg. Occasionally, smaller doses of each are administered however. The fibrates are used in patients with severe hyper-triglyceridemia in order to reduce the risk of pancreatitis. They are also used in patients with combined hyperlipidemia (frequently in combination with statins) to control the elevated triglyceride levels. However, there is no conclusive evidence that additional reductions in CHD risk occur beyond that obtained by LDL-C lowering alone, and there is an increased risk of myopathy. The VA-HIT trial results indicated that gemfibrozil is an option for therapy in patients with CHD who have LDL-C levels <130 mg/dL, together with low HDL.

THE SELECTION OF DRUGS AND INITIATION OF DRUG THERAPY

The primary focus for drug therapy is currently an elevated LDL-C, particularly in patients with additional risk factors. Subjects who are close to target goals may be given an initial trial of lifestyle and diet. However, patients who have CHD or CHD risk equivalents or require large reductions in LDL-C should have diet, lifestyle, and drug therapy initiated simultaneously. Secondary attention is given to HDL-C and triglyceride levels. Non-HDL-C (total-cholesterol – HDL-C) is recommended as a secondary target if triglycerides are >200 mg/dL. Significant reductions in triglyceride levels can frequently be achieved with diet, lifestyle and control of secondary causes, making drug therapy unnecessary. The current suggested guidelines for drug therapy from the NCEP[14] are discussed in Chapter 11 and summarized in Table 8.2.

Table 8.2 *Treatment targets for drug therapy (mg/dL)*

	Treatment goals (mg/dL)	
	LDL-C	Non-HDL-C*
CHD or CHD risk equivalent	<100	<130
Without CHD, ≥2 risk factors and 10-year risk <20%	<130	<160
Without CHD and 0–1 risk factors	<160	<190

*Non-HDL-cholesterol = Total cholesterol – HDL-cholesterol.

The NCEP guidelines were revised and reported in 2001[14] (see also Chapter 11). One major change is that absolute risk at baseline is now used to determine the intensity of LDL-C management. A new definition is CHD risk equivalent, which indicates a 10-year risk of fatal or non-fatal MI according to Framingham data of >20 percent in 10 years.[14] CHD risk equivalents include patients with clinical evidence of atherosclerotic disease in any arterial bed, diabetes mellitus, or two risk factors and 10-year risk of >20 percent. A secondary target of non-HDL-C is recommended for patients with triglyceride levels >200 mg/dL. The target level is 30 points higher than that for LDL-C. Drug therapy should be initiated in patients with acute coronary events before hospital discharge. The rationale is to improve endothelial function and plaque stabilization as quickly as possible, and there is also evidence that long-term compliance is better. The MIRACL trial demonstrated that atorvastatin at high dose (80 mg) decreased repeat hospitalizations for unstable angina with initiation of drug therapy prior to hospital discharge in patients with acute coronary syndrome.[15] The results of the follow-up to the Post-CABG study indicated that an LDL-C target goal of <100 mg/dL resulted in less progression and fewer coronary events than a mean LDL-C of 135 mg/dL.[7] There was still disagreement regarding the need for LDL-C lowering in CHD patients with LDL-C of 100–129 mg/dL. The VA-HIT study demonstrated a definite benefit in the group treated with gemfibrozil, whilst the Heart Protection Study[6] demonstrated significant benefit even in patients with LDL-C <100 mg/dL treated with a statin. Thus, it appears that all patients with CHD or CHD risk equivalents should receive drug therapy.

The amount of LDL-C lowering that is necessary to achieve target LDL-C goals is given in Table 8.3. The results of recent trials suggest that target levels considerably less than 100 mg/dL may be recommended for high-risk patients in the future. Also, the reported mean reductions in LDL-C that can be expected from the usual starting and maximum doses of currently approved statins are given in Table 8.4. The specific reduction in LDL-C obtainable in an individual patient can vary considerably from the population mean, but can generally be used to help select the specific statin or dose that will generally be required. In addition to many eligible patients not receiving any lipid-lowering drug therapy, another major problem is that the drug dosage is not titrated. Thus, a high percentage of patients are continued on their starting dose of statin. The data presented in Table 8.4 indicate that a large percentage of patients would not be expected to achieve the desired target LDL-C level with the recommended starting dose of many statins; many patients will not achieve target levels, even with the maximum dose of a number of statins.

Table 8.3 *Achieving target LDL-cholesterol (LDL-C) goals*

Baseline LDL-C (% reduction to achieve target goals)	130	160	190	220
Target LDL-C <100	24	38	48	55
Target LDL-C <130	–	19	32	41
Target LDL-C <160	–	–	16	28

Table 8.4 *Mean percentage reduction in LDL-cholesterol (LDL-C) with usual starting and maximum statin dose**

Statin	Starting dose		Maximum dose	
	mg	%∴LDL–C	mg	%∴LDL–C
Lovastatin	20	24	80	40
Pravastatin	20	24	80	40
Simvastatin	20	35	80	46
Fluvastatin	20	18	80	31
Fluvastatin (XL)	–	–	80	38
Atorvastatin	10	37	80	57

*Maximum dose currently approved by the FDA.

Combination therapy

The general approach to the selection of combination therapy in patients who have not achieved target LDL-C goals or who have multiple lipoprotein abnormalities is given in Table 8.5. The data in this table assume that patients began with elevated LDL-C levels at baseline, and that statin therapy has already been initiated.

Table 8.5 *Combination therapy if target goals are not achieved with statin therapy[a]*

Therapy	Reduce LDL-C	Increase HDL-C	Decrease triglycerides
Resin	1	3	–
Nicotinic acid	2	1	2
Fibrates	3	2	1

[a]Priorities are established based upon expected efficacy. Other factors may be considered.

SPECIFIC DISORDERED LIPID PATTERNS

Elevated LDL-C and triglycerides <200 mg/dL

Statins are the preferred initial drug. If only modest reductions in LDL-C are required, then resins and nicotinic acid can be considered, but these two classes of drugs are frequently not well tolerated. On average, an additional 6 percent lowering of LDL-C is obtained with each doubling of the dose of statin. Factors such as cost and side effects must be considered in deciding whether to go to maximum levels of statins or combination therapy to achieve target LDL-C goals. Resins are usually the most effective class for achieving additional LDL-C lowering in patients receiving a statin. The additional effect of resin therapy is not always predictable however, and the potential benefit should be evaluated clinically. Generally, the additional lowering of LDL-C with resin therapy will be less if the patient is already on maximum statin therapy as compared with lower statin dosages. Nicotinic acid can also be used for additional LDL-C lowering, but is usually used if HDL-C raising or lowering of triglyceride or Lp(a) levels are desired. In the past, nicotinic acid was also considered if administration of a tablet was desired. Resins are now available in tablet form (colesevelam, colestipol). If patients do not achieve target goals or do not tolerate the other three classes of drugs, then fenofibrate should be considered and some patients will achieve moderate LDL-C lowering. Triple drug therapy is occasionally required to achieve target goals, but this therapy may be complex and the alternative of referral to a specialized center should be considered. Rarely, LDL-apheresis is required.

Elevated LDL-C and triglycerides (combined hyperlipidemia)

These patients are characterized by elevated levels of LDL-C, triglycerides and triglyceride-rich particles, low HDL-C levels and smaller, more dense LDL particles.

Additionally, many of these patients are obese with abdominal obesity and insulin resistance and sometimes frank diabetes mellitus. Statins are usually the drugs of first choice; these reduce the concentration of all the atherogenic particles and increase HDL-C levels moderately. Some confusion has been generated because they may not convert the small dense LDL particles (Pattern B) to the larger LDL particles (Pattern A). However, the total number of particles – especially the small dense ones – is decreased. Clinical trial data have confirmed that LDL-C lowering reduces risk and should be the initial target for therapy. Generally, nicotinic acid or fibrates are then added to achieve control of HDL-C and triglyceride levels.

Nicotinic acid can be considered as initial therapy, especially if the required LDL-C lowering is modest. Nicotinic acid also favorably affects all of the atherogenic lipoprotein particles.[16] Concerns relate to the possibility of increased insulin resistance in patients who are either diabetic or prediabetic. This could decrease the benefits on CHD risk reduction. The findings of a recent study suggested that nicotinic acid in doses up to 3 g per day did not cause significant deterioration of glucose control in diabetic patients. However, there are still concerns about using nicotinic acid (especially at higher doses) in patients who have or who are prone to developing diabetes mellitus. The use of nicotinic acid in moderate doses primarily for increasing HDL-C levels and lowering triglycerides and triglyceride-rich particles is generally preferred.

Fibrates are generally used in combination with the statins, although there is an increased risk of myopathy. They are primarily effective in decreasing the concentrations of triglyceride and triglyceride-rich particles, but rarely achieve target LDL-C levels as monotherapy. The fibrates convert the small dense LDL particles to the larger LDL particles, and increases in total LDL-C levels are frequently seen with fibrate monotherapy. Fenofibrate is more effective in controlling LDL-C levels than gemfibrozil.

The omega-3 fatty acids do not appear to increase the risk of myopathy when co-administered with a statin. They are now being used more frequently for triglyceride lowering. At higher doses, there may be some risk of bleeding, and some patients dislike the taste. The dose is determined by titration and the severity of the triglyceride elevations. Daily doses in the range of 4–8 g are usually required.

Low HDL-C levels

Increasing HDL-C levels has not been shown conclusively to reduce CHD risk, though there is strong evidence from the VA-HIT trial that there is some benefit. If LDL-C levels are 130 mg/dL, the initial therapy is LDL-C lowering. The greatest benefit from lowering LDL-C levels has been demonstrated in patients with low HDL-C levels. In the VA-HIT trial, patients with LDL-C levels of <130 mg/dL, low HDL-C levels (mean 32 mg/dL) and modest increases in triglycerides who were treated with gemfibrozil had significant reductions in the risk of non-fatal MI, CHD death, and stroke. Most clinicians still favor statin therapy in this population, although some prefer fibrates as the initial drug.

Elevated triglycerides

When triglyceride levels are >400 mg/dL, there is no simple clinical test for quantifying LDL-C levels as neither direct measurement nor ultracentrifugation is frequently unavailable. Unless total cholesterol levels are very high, triglyceride-lowering therapy can be initiated, and the LDL-C levels can be evaluated later. Generally, when triglyceride levels are >750–1000 mg/dL the greatest concern is pancreatitis, whereas with levels under 500 mg/dL the concern is risk for CHD. Individuals with triglyceride levels between 500 and 750 mg/dL may have an increased risk for both CHD or pancreatitis, whereas patients with triglyceride levels of >750 mg/dL generally have elevated chylomicron levels. The two preferred therapies for lowering chylomicron levels are fibrates and omega-3 fatty acids which can be used either singly or in combination. Secondary causes of hyper-triglyceridemia must also be ruled out and corrected. Doses of omega-3 fatty acids in the range of 6–12 g/day may be necessary, depending upon the severity of the hypertriglyceridemia.

SUMMARY

Drug therapy has been shown conclusively to reduce CHD risk with all four major classes of lipid-lowering drugs that are currently available. Aggressive control of lipids and lipoproteins has been shown to reduce the clinical manifestation of the atherosclerotic process in all arterial beds. Statins are usually the drugs of first choice because the primary target of therapy is to control LDL-C levels. The currently suggested target goals of the National Cholesterol Education Program can now be achieved in almost all patients with a combination of diet, lifestyle, and drug therapy. Many patients can achieve their target goals with monotherapy, though some may require either combination or triple drug therapy to achieve this aim. Complex drug regimens may be facilitated by referral to a specialized center.

REFERENCES

1. Jones P, Kafonek S, Laurora I, Hunninghake D, for the CURVES Investigators. Comparative dose efficacy study of atorvastatin versus simvastatin, pravastatin, lovastatin and fluvastatin in patients with hypercholesterolemia (The CURVES study). *Am J Cardiol* 1998; **81**: 582–7.
2. Campeau L, Hunninghake DB, Knatterud GL, White CW, Domanski M, Forman SA, Forrester JS, Geller NL, Gobel FL, Herd JA, Hoogwerf BJ, Rosenberg Y for the Post CABG Trial Investigators. Aggressive cholesterol lowering delays saphenous vein graft atherosclerosis in women, in the elderly, and patients with associated risk factors: NHLBI Post Coronary Artery Bypass Graft Clinical Trial. *Circulation* 1999; **99**: 3241–7.
3. Bauer DC, Mundy GR, Jamel SA, *et al.* Statin use, bone mass and fracture: an analysis of two prospective studies. *J Bone Miner Res* 1999; **14** (Suppl. 1): S179.
4. Davidson MH. Does differing metabolism by cytochrome P450 have clinical importance? *Curr Atheroscler Reports* 2000; **2**: 14–19.

5. LaRosa JC, He J, Vupputuri S. Effect of statins on risk of coronary disease: a meta-analysis of randomized controlled trials. *JAMA* 1999; **282**: 2340–6.
6. Collins R, Armitage J, Parish S, Sleight P, Peto R for the Heart Protection Study Collaborative Group. MRC/BHF heart protection study of cholesterol lowering with simvastatin in 20,536 high-risk individuals: a randomised placebo-controlled trial. *Lancet* 2002; **360**: 7–22.
7. Campeau L, Knatterud GL, Domanski M, Hunninghake DB, White CW, Geller NL, Rosenberg Y for the Post Coronary Artery Bypass Graft Trial Investigators. The effect of aggressive lowering of low-density lipoprotein cholesterol levels and low-dose anticoagulation on obstructive changes in saphenous-vein coronary-artery bypass grafts. *N Engl J Med* 1997; **336**: 153–62.
8. Haffner SM, Alexander CM, Cook TJ, Boccuzzi SJ, Musliner TA, Pedersen TR, Kjekshus J, Pyorala K. Reduced coronary events in simvastatin-treated patients with coronary heart disease and diabetes or impaired fasting glucose levels: subgroup analyses in the Scandinavian Simvastatin Survival Study. *Arch Intern Med* 1999; **159**: 2661–7.
9. Davidson MH, Dillon MA, Gordon B, Jones P, Samuels J, Weiss S, Isaacsohn J, Toth P, Burke SK. Colesevelam hydrochloride (cholestagel): a new, potent bile acid sequestrant associated with a low incidence of gastrointestinal side effects. *Arch Intern Med* 1999; **159**: 1893–900.
10. Lipid Research Clinics Program. The Coronary Primary Prevention Trial Results, I: reduction in incidence of coronary heart disease. *JAMA* 1984; **251**: 351–64.
11. Canner PL, Berge KG, Wenger NK, *et al.* for the Coronary Drug Project Research Group. Fifteen year mortality in coronary drug project patients: long-term benefit with niacin. *J Am Coll Cardiol* 1986; **8**: 1245–55.
12. Frick MH, Elo O, Haapa K, *et al.* Helsinki Heart study: primary prevention trial with gemfibrozil in middle aged men with dyslipidemia: safety of treatment, changes in risk factors, and incidence of coronary heart disease. *N Engl J Med* 1987; **317**: 1237–45.
13. Rubins HB, Rubins SJ, Collins D, *et al.* Gemfibrozil for the secondary prevention of coronary heart disease in men with low levels of high-density lipoprotein cholesterol. Veterans Administration Affairs High-Density Lipoprotein Cholesterol Intervention Trial Study Group. *N Engl J Med* 1999; **341**: 401–18.
14. National Cholesterol Education Program Guidelines Adult Treatment Panel III (ATP III). (Summary form). *JAMA* 2001: **285**: 2486–97.
15. Schwartz GG, Olsson AG, Ezekowitz, *et al.* Effects of atorvastatin on early recurrent ischemic events in acute coronary syndromes. *JAMA* 2001; **285**: 1711–18.
16. Guyton JR, Blazing MA, Hagar J, Kashyap ML, Knopp RH, McKenney JM, Nash DT, Nash SD. Extended-release niacin vs. gemfibrozil for the treatment of low levels of high-density lipoprotein cholesterol – Niaspan-Gemfibrozil Study Group. *Arch Intern Med* 2000; **160**: 1177–84.

9

Costs of lipid-lowering therapy with statins

MICHAEL D KLEIN

INTRODUCTION

A standard definition of healthcare cost might be an amount paid or required in payment for purchase of a service. That service might entail a doctor's office visit, or the performance of a laboratory test, or the consumption of medication. Increasingly, however, healthcare costs have extended beyond the well-being of an individual and encompass social, economic, and political concerns. Viewed from these perspectives, ancillary definitions of cost as a burden, loss, or penalty have taken on added importance in the struggle to constrain healthcare expenditures.

Several agencies and numerous strategies have been proposed for managing healthcare costs, and these are summarized in Boxes 9.1 and 9.2. In the case of drug expenditures – especially those given over protracted time intervals to treat chronic illnesses – physician-oriented policies to restrain costs and enhance the efficiency drug usage have been reviewed.[1] Budgetary restrictions, dissemination of information on prescribing analysis and cost, and prescription guidelines are three mechanisms widely used by government and, to a lesser extent, industry to curb drug expenditures. Rigorous evaluation of the cost savings and, more cogently, the cost-effectiveness of these measures over the long as well as the short term, has not been completed, however. Indeed, recommendations for standardizing the reporting of cost-effective analyses have only recently been proposed.[2]

Box 9.1   *Agencies for limiting drug costs*

Budgetary limitations
    Government
        National
        Regional
    Industry
        Pharmaceutical companies
        Managed healthcare companies
    Health professions
        Hospitals
        Physicians
        Pharmacy management

Box 9.2   *Strategies for limiting drug costs*

Global budget setting
    Inflation, demographics, epidemiological adjustments
        New scientific advances
Hospital/physician incentives
    Financial awards or penalties
Practice guidelines
Marketplace competition
Pharmacoeconomic data
    Cost minimization studies
    Cost-effectiveness studies

The therapeutic value of various pharmaceutical interventions has been codified within clinical practice guidelines which have graded the quality of evidence that various drug treatments achieve their desired therapeutic effects and influenced outcome.[3] Such methods employ evidence-based medicine to distinguish amongst probably effective, possibly effective, and questionably effective drug treatment algorithms.[4] A more refined version of drug efficacy combines the evidence from clinical assessment with formal cost-effectiveness analyses.[5] The combined approach is applicable to both secondary and primary prevention and may result in enhanced benefits as, for example, the screening for asymptomatic hypothyroidism by screening individuals for both thyroid-stimulating hormone and cholesterol levels.[6]

While elevated serum cholesterol can suggest occult hypothyroidism, its presence denotes an increased risk for coronary heart disease (CHD) and a suitable target for risk factor intervention. A systematic review of 28 randomized trials of cholesterol lowering with drugs and diet indicated that a 10 percent lowering of cholesterol resulted in a 10 percent reduction in coronary mortality and an 18 percent reduction in coronary events. The importance of sustained cholesterol lowering was even more striking. Maintaining drug treatment for 5 years reduced the coronary event rate by

25 percent when observational studies were combined with randomized clinical trials.[7] Correcting for regression dilution bias (variation in cholesterol levels over time) and surrogate dilution bias [closer correlation of low-density lipoprotein (LDL) than total cholesterol with coronary event rate] suggests that a 10 percent cholesterol increase translates into a 28 percent increment in CHD risk.[8]

COSTS OF SECONDARY PREVENTION

Clinical trial data utilizing more potent cholesterol-lowering drugs have shown even greater benefits. For secondary prevention, statin drugs manifested a 24–42 percent reduction in relative risk for coronary events, and significant reductions in the need for re-hospitalization and need for coronary interventional procedures, percutaneous transluminal coronary angiography (PTCA), and coronary artery bypass grafting (CABG) surgery.[9,10]

More recent sub-group analyses from the Scandinavian Simvastatin Survival Study (4S) and Cholesterol and Recurrent Events (CARE) study populations[11,12] have generated controversy regarding the optimal goals for LDL lowering in secondary prevention which current National Cholesterol Education Program (NCEP) Guidelines[13] stipulate as ≤100 mg/dL. Three models have been proposed to describe the effects of serum LDL-cholesterol (LDL-C) reduction on the relative risk for CHD: a linear relationship; a threshold relationship; and a curvilinear relationship.[14] Data from the largest cohort date of patients followed prospectively in the MRFIT Study indicated a curvilinear relationship[15] supporting the NCEP guideline approach of modulating the intensity of LDL-C lowering to the patient-specific absolute risk. Continual though diminishing coronary event reduction might be anticipated, with total cholesterol lowering to 160 mg/dL or LDL-C lowering to 75–80 mg/dL, but such aggressive pharmacological therapy remains to be verified by further randomized trial data.

Several pharmacoeconomic studies with statins have been completed. A cost minimization analysis from prospectively collected data in the 4S study[16] indicated that simvastatin-treated patients had 34 percent reduced recurrent hospitalization days. When spread over the 5.4 years of the study, net cholesterol drug treatment costs were 28 cents per day, amortizing these statin drug costs by 88 percent.[12] Conversion of 4S study cost minimization data to cost-effectiveness analysis indicated that statin drug treatment for secondary coronary prevention would obviate a major cardiovascular event or death at a 5-year cost of $11 640 and $23 280, respectively. Individual patient costs and benefits depended upon the age at which treatment was initiated, the duration of treatment, and the presence and control of associated risk factors for coronary disease.

A 4S analysis which stratified for age, sex, and baseline cholesterol level prior to treatment and with separate estimates for men and women, at various ages of 35–70 years, and with total cholesterol levels of between 213 and 309 mg/dL has also been detailed.[17] Direct costs per year of life gained ranged from $3800 for a 70-year-old male with a serum cholesterol level of 309 mg/dL to $27 400 for a 35-year-old female with a serum cholesterol level of 213 mg/dL. If indirect costs were included, actual savings were computed for the youngest patients, and costs of $13 300 per year of life gained tallied for a 70-year-old woman with a serum cholesterol level of 213 mg/dL.

The cost-effectiveness of pravastatin in two placebo-controlled plaque regression clinical trials has also been modeled in the male cohort of 445 patients from the PLAC I and PLAC II studies.[18] Cost per life-year saved ranged from $7124 to $12 665 depending upon the number of prevailing risk factors in the coronary artery disease (CAD) males. This was consonant with the Harvard Risk Analysis Survey amongst 500 life-saving interventions, where the median cost per life-year saved for secondary prevention was about $19 000.[19] The available data from randomized statin drug trials commend this form of medical therapy, both from a clinical and an economic perspective.[20]

ANCILLARY ISSUES IN SECONDARY COST PREVENTION

The primary focus of statin randomized clinical trials has been the reduction of coronary events. Recent meta-analyses have also correlated a 30 percent lowering of LDL-C with a 29 percent risk reduction in stroke – a highly significant relative risk reduction of 0.76.[21,22] In the CARE study in post-myocardial infarction (MI) patients with moderately elevated LDL-cholesterol levels, pravastatin reduced stroke risk from 7.3 to 5.0 per 1000 patient-years (32%), with similar reductions in sub-group analyses defined by history of hypertension, diabetes, or prior stroke.[23] By comparison, stroke risk was reduced by 29 percent in the 4S study.[24] The ability of satin drugs to lower stroke risk in secondary prevention is disproportionately greater than for other classes of cholesterol-lowering agents,[25] and this may have a major impact in the future of lowering healthcare expenditures for what can be a chronically disabling and costly disease.

The mechanisms by which statin drugs might reduce stroke risk remain uncertain. Their anti-atherothrombotic properties have been commented upon,[26] and particularly their potential for promoting plaque stability, delimiting platelet reactivity, promoting fibrinolysis, and suppressing plaque thrombosis. Possible anti-oxidant properties and inhibition of smooth muscle migration have also been noted in a commentary on the mechanism whereby statins might reduce cardiovascular events by reducing plaque volume.[27] Evidence to support anti-inflammatory and immune-related properties of statins which might retard atherosclerotic progression[28] and thereby lower the long-term cost of patient care has also been noted.[28]

Costs of primary prevention

The cost-effectiveness of lipid drug treatment for primary prevention in coronary disease remains more controversial. Epidemiological and scientific data persuasively link elevated blood cholesterol levels to atherosclerosis and coronary events.[29,30] Economic concerns have been raised about the substantial drug costs engendered by treating such large numbers of asymptomatic individuals, however.[31] Economic and scientifically oriented perspectives have even resulted in clashing professional society clinical guidelines for drug use in treating hypercholesterolemia.[32–34] Evidence-based clinical trial data for individuals with very high cholesterol and LDL levels (272 and 192 mg/dL, respectively) indicate that statin treatment which lowers cholesterol by 20 percent reduces coronary event risk by 31 percent and mortality risk by 22 percent.[35] Questions linger, however, concerning the cost and cost-effectiveness of primary prevention for individuals with lower (though still elevated) serum cholesterol and LDL levels (200–250 mg/dL and 130–180 mg/dL, respectively). Life-table modeling of statin drug treatment over a 10-year interval in men and women, aged between 45 and 64 years, clearly portrays clinical efficacy and safety, but queries persist as to whether a purchasing authority could afford the estimated cost of $217 600 per life-year saved for primary prevention.[36]

Data from one AFCAPS/Tex CAPS study indicated that statin therapy significantly reduced the first major coronary event in a population followed for 5.2 years and composed of 5608 men and 997 women with a mean cholesterol of 221 mg/dL, LDL of 150 mg/dL, and high-density lipoprotein (HDL) of 36 mg/dL in men and 40 mg/dL in women.[37] The relative risk for MI and unstable angina was reduced to 0.60 and 0.68 respectively, while the number of coronary revascularization procedures required was reduced by about one-third. The cumulative reduction in hospitalization and cardiac interventional procedures would translate into consider-able cost savings but, as yet, no formal cost-minimalization or cost-effectiveness analyses have been performed in the AFCAPS/Tex CAPS population.

Time perspective

Overwhelming evidence links high cholesterol levels to atherosclerosis, vascular endothelial cell dysfunction, and coronary morbidity and mortality. Epidemiological studies indicate that adverse levels of LDL-C persist over time and progress to adult dyslipidemia, often accompanied by weight gain.[38] Cholesterol has also been established as being predictive of long-term CHD events over a 15- to 30-year prospective interval, and with little change in the strength of this association.[39–41] Might diet and exercise programs which entail no drug costs mitigate this problem? If short-term studies can be used as a guide, there is scant hope of this prospect. For example, a 1-year dietary intervention to prevent obesity and lower saturated fat and cholesterol intake achieved only a modest LDL-C reduction of 12 mg/dL which increased only slightly to 15 mg/dL with the addition of behavioral intervention. And while prevention education programs to reinforce nutritional health or enhance physical activity can achieve short-term enhancement of cardiorespiratory fitness[42] and possibly affect lifetime habits,[43] the longer-term impact of such initiatives on cardiovascular morbidity and mortality remains unknown. Moreover, are short-term dietary management schemes sustainable over longer time periods for the vast majority of individuals? Though structured office space or nutritional center counseling and surveillance with a Step I AHA Diet elicited a two- to four-fold improvement in cholesterol lowering compared with usual care, absolute reductions were still modest at 12 and 21 mg/dL, respectively.[44] Are these reductions however laudable and inexpensive in dollar costs quantitatively sufficient to impact coronary morbidity and mortality and achieve savings in preventive care?

The predisposition to atherosclerosis begins *in utero*, and is associated with hypercholesterolemia during pregnancy.[45] Both necropsy and epidemiological data confirm the association of elevated cholesterol and obesity with atherosclerosis in children and young adults.[46,47] While many physicians are still hesitant about using drugs to lower cholesterol in children at high risk for later life cardiovascular events, the results of recent studies have suggested that it is safe to lower dietary fat without harming growth during the first 3 years of childhood[48] or later in childhood.[49] Although data with statin drug therapy are still meager, a study of lovastatin in heterozygous familial hypercholesterolemic adolescent males, revealed no adverse affects on either growth or sexual development after 48 weeks of observation.[50] Therefore, a renewed effort to combat atherosclerosis in childhood seems clearly warranted, even in the absence of long-term pharmacoeconomic studies.[51]

FUTURE DIRECTIONS

The adage that short-term gains do not necessarily translate into long-term advantages has great relevance for coronary atherosclerosis – a disease that requires several decades to evolve. Societies and governments that are preoccupied with 'quick fixes' to medical problems as they happen often pay more for salvage and restitution than they would have had they extended effort and resources to prevent or at least retard the onset of these very same problems. Viewed from this perspective, the treatment of hypercholesterolemia – especially for primary prevention – will require a balancing of scientific and economic objectives; also, a willingness on the part of healthcare payors and regulators to pay now in order to save later, even if this means adding drug costs to dietary restraints; and, finally, an appreciation that an ounce of prevention requires both discipline and resolve.

The pharmacoeconomics of LDL cholesterol management[44] make a strong case for the use of statin drugs. Available randomized clinical trial data support the cost-effectiveness of this drug intervention strategy in all patients with an annual coronary event risk of >1 percent. For those with evidence of pre-existing athero-sclerotic vascular disease or diabetes, the risk reduction and the ensuing rewards – both clinical and economic – should be evident to physicians and health planners alike.

For patients with lower boundaries of risk and for primary prevention of cardio-vascular disease, statin therapy shows great promise and may lead to refinements in currently prevailing clinical guidelines.[52] Multiple risk factor appraisals[53] and computer-driven assessments of event risk will likely impact on clinical guidelines and usage patterns. Current iterations recommend lipid-lowering drug intervention when the 10-year coronary heart disease risk is either 20 percent or greater,[54] or a gradualist approach of risk beginning at >3 percent and extending down to 15 percent.[55]

One concern regarding randomized clinical trials is their relevance to the single patient in clinical practice.[56] Do the outcomes of the many in the study populations pertain to the unique clinical risk factor mix of a particular individual? One approach to minimizing any potential discrepancies will be the reporting of additional large randomized trials[57] undergoing the referral database.

Uncertainty also extends to data evaluation, and particularly in the case of a clinical outcome measure such as cost-effectiveness.[58] Standard statistical measures for applying boundaries (95% confidence intervals) around point estimates which cannot easily be applied to cost analyses are supplanted by one of several methods of sensitivity analytical techniques.

Given this background and a database from long-term population studies which distinguish between low- and high-risk patients,[59] cost-effectiveness in lipid management is likely to reflect a shifting balance of risk management, professional and political imperatives.[60]

REFERENCES

1. Bloor K, Freemantle N. Lessons from international experience in controlling pharmaceutical expenditure II: Influencing doctors. *Br Med J* 1996; **312**: 1525–7.
2. Siegel JE, Weinstein MC, Russell LB, Gold MR. For the panel on Cost Effectiveness in Health and Medicine. *JAMA* 1996; **276**: 1339–41.
3. US Preventive Services Task Force. *Guide To Clinical Preventive Services.* 2nd edition. Baltimore, MD: Williams & Wilkins; 1996.
4. ACC/AHA Practice Guidelines. Guidelines for the management of patients with acute myocardial infarction. *J Am Coll Cardiol* 1996; **28**: 1328–428.
5. Clancy CM, Karerow BV. Evidence-based medicine meets cost-effectiveness analysis. *JAMA* 1996; **276**: 329–30.
6. Danese MD, Powe MR, Swain CT, Ladenson PW. Screening for mild thyroid failure at the periodic health examination: a decision and cost-effectiveness analysis. *JAMA* 1996; **276**: 285–92.
7. Law MR, Wald NJ, Thompson SG. By how much and how quickly does reduction in serum cholesterol lower risk of ischemic heart disease. *Br Med J* 1994; **308**: 367–72.
8. Gaziano JM, Hebert PR, Hennekens CH. Cholesterol reduction: weighing the benefits and risks. *Ann Intern Med* 1996; **124**: 914–18.
9. Randomized trial of cholesterol lowering in 4,444 patients with coronary heart disease: The Scandinavian Simvastatin Survival Study (4S). *Lancet* 1994; **344**: 1383–9.
10. Sacks FM, Pfeffer MA, Moye LA, Rouleau JL, Rutherford JD, Cole TG, Braunwald EB. The effect of pravastatin on coronary events in myocardial infarction patients with average cholesterol levels. *N Engl J Med* 1996; **335**: 1001–9.
11. Pedersen TR, Olsson AG, Faergeman O, Kjekshus J, Wedel H, Berg K, Wilhelmsen L, Haghfeld D, Thorgeirsson G, Pyorala K, Miettinen T, Christophersen B, Tobert JA, Musliner TA, Cook TJ, for the Scandinavian Simvastatin Survival Study Group. Lipoprotein changes and reduction in the incidence of major coronary heart disease events in the Scandinavian Simvastatin Survival Study (4S). *Circulation* 1998; **97**: 1453–60.
12. Sacks FM, Moye LA, Davis BR, *et al.* Relationship between plasma LDL concentrations during treatment with pravastatin and recurrent coronary events in the Cholesterol and Recurrent Events trial. *Circulation* 1998; **97**: 1446–52.
13. Summary of the Second Report of the National Cholesterol Education Program (NCEP) Expert Panel on Detection, Evaluation, and Treatment of High Blood Cholesterol in Adults (Adult Treatment Panel II). *JAMA* 1993; **269**: 3015–23.

14. Grundy SM. Statin trials and the goals of cholesterol-lowering therapy. *Circulation* 1998; **97**: 1436–9.
15. Stamler J, Wentworth D, Neaton JB. Is the relationship between serum cholesterol and risk of premature death from coronary heart disease continuous and graded? Findings in 356,222 primary screenees of the Multiple Risk Factor Intervention Trial (MRFIT). *JAMA* 1986; **256**: 2823–8.
16. Pedersen TR, Kjekshus J, Berg K, *et al*. Scandinavian Simvastatin Survival Study. *Circulation* 1996; **93**: 1792–802.
17. Johannesson M, Jonsson B, Kjekshus J, Olsson AG, Pedersen TR, Wedel H. Cost-effectiveness of simvastatin treatment of lower cholesterol levels in patients with coronary heart disease. *N Engl J Med* 1997; **336**: 332–6.
18. Ashraf T, Hay JW, Pitt B, Wittels E, Crouse J, Davidson M, Furberg CD, Redican L. Cost-effectiveness of pravastatin in secondary prevention of coronary artery disease. *Am J Cardiol* 1996; **78**: 409–14.
19. Szucs TD. Pharmaco-economic aspects of lipid-lowering therapy: is it worth the price? *Eur Heart J* 1998; **19** (Suppl.): M22–8.
20. Tengs TO, Adams ME, Pliskin AS, *et al*. Five hundred lifesaving interventions and their cost-effectiveness. *Risk Analysis* 1995; **15**: 369–90.
21. Hebert PR, Gaziano JM, Chan KS, Hennekens CH. Cholesterol lowering with statin drug, risk of stroke and total mortality: an overview of randomized trials. *JAMA* 1997; **278**: 313–21.
22. Bucher HC, Griffith LE, Guyatt GH. Effect of NMG Let reductase inhibitors on stroke: a meta-analysis of randomized, controlled trials. *Ann Intern Med* 1998; **128**: 89–95.
23. Plehn JF, David BR, Sachs FM, *et al*. Reduction of stroke evidence after myocardial infarction with pravastatin. *Circulation* 1999; **99**: 216–33.
24. Pederson TR, Kjekshus J, Pyorala K, *et al*. Effect of simvastatin on ischemic stroke victims in the Scandinavian Simvastatin Survival Study (4-S). *Am J Cardiol* 1998; **81**: 333–5.
25. Rosenderff C. Statins for the prevention of stroke. *Lancet* 1998; **351**: 1002–3.
26. Rosenson MD, Tangney CC. Antiatherothrombotic properties of statins: implications for cardiovascular event reduction. *JAMA* 1998; **279**: 1643–50.
27. Archbald RA, Timmis AD. Cholesterol lowering and coronary artery disease: mechanism of risk reduction. *Heart* 1998; **80**: 543–7.
28. Vaughan CJ, Murphy MB, Buckley BM. Statins do more than just lower cholesterol. *Lancet* 1996; **348**: 1079–82.
29. Yusuf S. Cost of prevention. The case of lipid lowering. *Circulation* 1996; **93**: 1774–6.
30. LaRosa JC. Cholesterol agonists. *Ann Intern Med* 1996; **124**: 1505–8.
31. Gafni A. Economic evaluation of healthcare interventions: an economist's perspective. *Am Coll Phys J Club* 1996; **124**: 12–A14.
32. Clinical Guidelines, Part I. Guidelines for using serum cholesterol, high-density lipoprotein cholesterol, and triglyceride levels as screening tests for preventing coronary heart disease in adults. American College of Physicians. *Ann Intern Med* 1996; **124**: 515–17.
33. Garber AM, Browner WS, Hully SB. Clinical guidelines, Part II. Cholesterol screening in asymptomatic adults, revisited. *Ann Intern Med* 1996; **124**: 518–31.
34. Cholesterol screening in asymptomatic adults. No cause to change. Task Force on Risk Reduction, American Heart Association. *Circulation* 1996; **93**: 1067–8.
35. Shepherd J, Cobbe SM, Ford I, Isles CG, Lorimer AR, MacFarlane PW, McKillop JH, Packard CJ for the West of Scotland Coronary Prevention Study Group. Prevention of coronary heart

disease with pravastatin in men with hypercholesterolemia. *N Engl J Med* 1995; **333**: 1301–7.

36. Pharoah PBP, Hollingworth HW. Cost effectiveness of lowering cholesterol concentration with statins in patients with and without pre-existing coronary heart disease: life table method applied to health authority population. *Br Med J* 1996; **312**: 1443–8.

37. Beere PA, Langendorfer A, Stein EA, Kruyer W, Gotte AM, Jr for the AFCAPS/TexCAPS Research Group. Primary prevention of acute coronary events with lovastatin in men and women with average cholesterol levels. Results of the AFCAPS/TexCAPS. *JAMA* 1998; **279**: 1615–22.

38. Bao W, Srinvasan SR, Wattigney MS, Berenson GS. Usefulness of childhood low-density lipoprotein cholesterol level in predicting adult dyslipidemia and cardiovascular risks. The Bogaulusa Heart Study. *Arch Intern Med* 1996; **156**: 1315–20.

39. Welin L, Eriksson H, Larsson B, *et al*. Risk factors for coronary heart disease during 25 years of follow-up. *Cardiology* 1993; **82**: 223–8.

40. Pekkanen J, Tervahauta M, Wissinen A, *et al*. Does the predictive value of baseline coronary risk factor change over a 30-year follow-up. *Cardiology* 1993; **82**: 181–90.

41. Wannamethel SG, Shaper AG, Whincup PH, Walker M. Role of risk factors for major coronary heart disease events with increasing length of follow-up. *Heart* 1999; **81**: 374–9.

42. Dunn AL, Marcus BH, Kampert JB, Garcia MF. Kehl HW, III, Blair SN. Comparison of lifestyle and structured interventions to increase physical activity and cardiorespiratory fitness: a randomized trial. *JAMA* 1999; **281**: 327–34.

43. Schwandt P, Geiss HC, Rotter MM, Ublocker C, Parhofer KG, Lamback OC, Donner MG, Hass GM, Richter WO. The Prevention Education Program (PEP). A prospective study of the reduction of family-oriented life style modification in the reduction of cardiovascular risk and disease: design and baseline data. *J Clin Epidemiol* 1999; **52**: 791–800.

44. Hay JW, Yu WM, Ashraf T. Pharmacoeconomics of lipid-lowering agents for primary and secondary prevention of coronary artery disease. *Pharmacoeconomics* 1999; **15**: 47–74.

45. Napoli C, Glass CK, Witzlum JL, Deutsch R, D'Armientio P, Palinski W. Influence of maternal hypercholesterolemia during pregnancy on the progression of early atherosclerotic lesions in childhood: Fate of Early Lesions in Children (FELIC) study. *Lancet* 1999; **354**: 1234–41.

46. Relationship of atherosclerosis in young men to serum lipoprotein cholesterol concentration and smoking: a preliminary report from the Pathobiological Determinants of Atherosclerosis in Youth (PDAY) Research Group. *JAMA* 1990; **264**: 3018–24.

47. Berenson GS, Wattigney WA, Tracy RE, *et al*. Atherosclerosis of the aortic and coronary arteries and cardiovascular risk factors in patients aged 6-30 years and studied at necropsy (The Bogalusa Heart Study). *Am J Cardiol* 1992; **70**: 851–8.

48. Niinkowski H, Lapinleimn H, Viikari J, *et al*. Growth until 3 years of age in a prospective randomized trial of diet with reduced saturated fat and cholesterol. *Pediatrics* 1997; **99**: 687–94.

49. DISC Collaborative Research Group. Efficacy and safety of lowering dietary intake of fat and cholesterol in children with elevated low density lipoprotein cholesterol. *JAMA* 1995; **273**: 1429–35.

50. Stein EA, Illingworth DR, Kwiterovich PO, *et al*. Efficacy and safety of lovastatin in adolescent males with heterozygous familial hypercholesterolemia: a randomized controlled trial. *JAMA* 1999; **281**: 137–44.

51. Berenson GS, Srinivasan SR. Prevention of atherosclerosis in children. *Lancet* 1999; **354**: 1223–4.

52. Pearson TA. Lipid-lowering therapy in low risk patients. *JAMA* 1998; **279**: 1659–61.
53. Anderson KM, Wilson PWF, Odell PM, Kannel UB. An updated coronary risk profile: a statement for health professionals. *Circulation* 1991; **83**: 356–62.
54. Wood D, DeBacker C, Faergemann O, *et al*. Prevention of coronary heart disease in clinical practice: recommendations of the Second Joint Task Force of Joint European Societies on Coronary Prevention. *Eur Heart J* 1998; **19**: 1434–503.
55. British Cardiac Society, British Hyperlipidaemia Association, British Hypertension Society [Endorsed by the British Diabetic Association]. Joint British Recommendations on the Prevention of Coronary Heart Disease in Clinical Practice. *Heart* 1998; **80** (Suppl. 2): S1–32.
56. Mant D. Evidence and primary care: can randomized trials uniform clinical decisions about individual patients? *Lancet* 1999; **353**: 743–6.
57. Prevention of cardiovascular events and death with pravastatin in patients with coronary heart disease and a broad range of initial cholesterol levels. The Long-Term Intervention with Pravastatin in Ischemic Disease (LIPID) Study Group. *N Engl J Med* 1998; **339**: 1349–57.
58. Briggs A. Handling uncertainty in economic evaluation. *Br Med J* 1999; **319**: 120–2.
59. Wilson PWF, D'Agestino RB, Levy D, Belanger AM, Silbershatz H, Kammel UB. Prediction of coronary heart disease using risk factor categories. *Circulation* 1998; **97**: 1837–47.
60. Grover S. Gambling with cardiovascular risk: picking the winners and the losers. *Lancet* 1999; **353**: 254.

10

Practical issues in implementation of lipid management

MERLE MYERSON

INTRODUCTION

There is a growing knowledge base, both in clinical trials and basic science, that supports the practice of lipid lowering. This evidence was reviewed in Chapter 1 and includes the pathophysiology, molecular biology, epidemiology, and economic aspects that demonstrate the benefits of treating hyperlipidemia.

Guidelines for risk factor reduction in general – and lipid lowering in particular – have been established, most notably the National Cholesterol Education Program and the Adult treatment Panel II and III (NCEP ATP II and III) Guidelines (see Chapter 11). However, clinicians have fallen short of implementing these recommendations: data from NHANES III show the magnitude of the potential problem. Almost 32 percent of adults surveyed required low-density lipoprotein-cholesterol (LDL-C) reduction.[1] Data from different populations, both in the United States and in Europe, further demonstrate the gap in management of lipid abnormalities.

Extent of undertreatment, and barriers to implementation of lipid management

Sempos and colleagues applied NCEP-ATP II guidelines to data from NHANES II and concluded that approximately 36 percent of US adults aged between 20 and 74 years need treatment for high blood cholesterol.[2] Giles *et al.* estimated the proportion of persons who need treatment based on NCEP-ATP guidelines and were receiving therapy.[3] These authors found that only about 28 percent of those who need treatment receive it; furthermore men, individuals aged between 20 and 39 years, and also blacks less often received treatment. In their data, Giles also found that among the 126 571 persons who had a physician visit in the previous 2 years for preventive care, 39.6 percent reported not being screened for cholesterol. Those missed were more likely to be black, Hispanic, aged between 20 and 39, and with less than 12 years of education.[3] Estimates of the number of subjects who would require drug therapy under the latest ATP III guidelines has tripled.

Among 90 patients who had received hexamethylglutaryl-coenzyme A (HMG-CoA) reductase inhibitors for 1 year, only 33 percent met their LDL-cholesterol goal.[4] However, only two patients who did not reach this goal were on maximum doses of drug, and most were not in the process of having their treatment plan adjusted. Compliance and cost (medications at the VA hospital were at no charge or nominal charge) were not felt to account for these findings.

In the Rural Lipid Resource Center Study of 16 primary care practices in Upstate New York, 307 patients were followed after their detection of blood cholesterol levels of 200 mg/dL or greater in 1992–93.[5] For those patients with no coronary disease and fewer than two risk factors ($n = 97$), 60.8 percent had reached their LDL-C goal of <160 mg/dL by 9 months. In contrast, of those patients without coronary heart disease (CHD) but with two or more risk factors ($n = 44$), only 9 percent had reached their LDL-C goal of 130 mg/dL. Most disconcerting were the 53 patients with CHD, as at the end of 9 months none had reached their goal of <100 mg/dL. Over 60 percent of the high-risk patients and over 80 percent of the CHD patients were

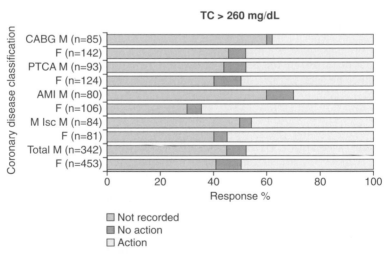

Figure 10.1 *Response as noted in the medical records of patients from the ASPIRE Study with total cholesterol (TC)≥260 mg/dL.[6] Response actions include: not recorded; no action; or action. Population divided by sex and coronary disease category, coronary artery bypass grafting (CABG), percutaneous transluminal coronary angioplasty (PTCA), acute myocardial infarction (AMI) or myocardial ischemia. M Isc: myocardial ischemia without AMI.*

candidates for cholesterol-lowering drug therapy according to National Cholesterol Education Program (NCEP) guidelines 9 months after initiation of dietary therapy. However, only 3 percent of high-risk and only 9 percent of CHD patients had been prescribed these agents.

Prevalence of non-treatment outside the United States is evident from the ASPIRE study. This trial enrolled 2583 coronary disease patients from 12 specialty hospitals and 12 district general hospitals in the United Kingdom (ASPIRE Steering Group).[6] Patient records frequently had no recording of risk factors, suggesting that no effort had been made to identify risk factors. In a small minority, risk factors were assessed but not acted upon. Approximately 50 percent of patients with body mass indices of >30 kg/m², blood glucose levels of 10 mmol/L, or systolic blood pressures of >160 mmHg, had any action taken. For patients with total cholesterol levels >260 mg/dL (6.5 mmol/L), the proportion of patients receiving any further action was also approximately 50 percent, and this did not differ much by sex or by category or coronary disease (Figure 10.1). In these high-risk patients, the prevalence of use of pharmacotherapies with proven efficacy to prevent recurrence and death was low at 6 months after discharge (Table 10.1).[6]

The objective of this chapter is first to identify the barriers to implementation that exist at various levels: patient-related factors, those involving physicians, organizational issues within the healthcare setting, and societal factors. Following this, strategies to improve implementation will be discussed. This includes interventions by physicians, allied health professionals, institutions, and healthcare systems. The role of pharmaceutical companies in developing and making available medications will also be addressed. Finally, recommendations for enactment of these strategies and for further research will be discussed. The barriers to implementation of preventive services at several different levels are listed in Box 10.1.[7]

Table 10.1 *Percentage of patients receiving drug therapy 6 months after discharge from hospitalization for coronary artery disease, by sex and diagnostic category in the ASPIRE study*[6]

Diagnostic Category	Sex	β–blocker	ACE inhibitor	Lipid–lowering therapy
CABG	M	18	17	18
	F	25	18	29
PTCA	M	43	13	18
	F	50	10	23
Myocardial ischemia	M	35	28	6
	F	41	24	10
AMI	M	39	20	9
	F	37	13	11

AMI: acute myocardial infarction; ASPIRE: Action in Secondary Prevention Through Intervention to Reduce Events; CABG: coronary artery bypass grafting; PTCA: percutaneous transluminal coronary angioplasty.

Box 10.1   *Barriers to implementation of preventive services*[7]

Patient
>   Lack of knowledge and motivation
>   Lack of access to care
>   Cultural factors
>   Social factors

Physician
>   Problem-based focus
>   Feedback on prevention is negative or neutral
>   Time constraints
>   Lack of incentives, including reimbursement
>   Lack of training
>>   Poor knowledge of benefits
>>   Perceived ineffectiveness
>>   Lack of skills
>   Lack of specialist–generalist communication
>   Lack of perceived legitimacy

Healthcare settings (hospitals, practices, etc.)
>   Acute care priority
>   Lack of resources and facilities
>   Lack of systems for preventive services

Time and economic constraints

Poor communication between specialist and primary care providers

Lack of policies and standards

Community/society
>   Lack of policies and standards
>   Lack of reimbursement

EXISTENCE OF BARRIERS AT DIFFERENT LEVELS

Patient factors

Kottke and colleagues have described patient demand as being the most powerful determinant of whether a physician addresses a patient's problem.[8] This perceived lack of patient motivation to initiate preventive care or adherence to preventive practices impedes delivery of these services.

Of those patients who are treated, non-compliance with treatment plan is another barrier. Simons and colleagues evaluated discontinuation rates in patients recently prescribed lipid-lowering drugs.[9] These authors reviewed 12 months' dispensing data in community pharmacies and found that a large proportion of discontinuations were patient-initiated; the reason cited was that the patient was not convinced of the need for ongoing, lifelong treatment. Rates for discontinuation vary. Andrade and colleagues found that rates in a Health Maintenance Organization (HMO) were substantially higher than reported in randomized clinical trials.[10] Bile acid sequestrants were discontinued at a rate of 41 percent in HMOs versus 31 percent in randomized trials. For niacin, these values were 46 percent and 4 percent, respectively. Rates for gemfibrozil were 37 percent versus 15 percent.[10] Enrollees in the New Jersey Medicaid and pharmacy assistance program for the aged and disabled and Quebec's provincial medical care program were followed for the proportion of time that they had filled their prescriptions. Overall, patients failed to fill prescriptions for lipid-lowering drugs for about 40 percent of the time.[11]

Schectman and Hiatt examined the extent that lipid goals were achievable in clinical practice.[12] While 75 percent of cardiovascular disease patients with an LDL ≤160 mg/dL achieved their goal with drug therapy, less than half of those with LDL >160 mg/dL did so. Patients who reported poor adherence to a medical regimen were less likely to achieve goals. The cumulative discontinuance rate for niacin and/or bile acid sequestrants was over 50 percent. While statins are generally regarded to have fewer side effects, the authors point out that patients with more severe elevations of cholesterol will often need combination therapy, so other drugs will remain important.

There is a tendency to fault the patient for failure to comply with a treatment regimen. Because coronary artery disease is a chronic disease, either chronic or long-term therapy is required. Without sustained intervention – both behavioral and therapeutic – successful risk reduction will be difficult to attain. However, there are external factors that influence patients' ability to participate in their own medical care. Strong associations have been demonstrated between indices of lower socio-economic status and a poor prognosis after diagnosis of CHD.[13,14] Many studies have examined racial differences in the prognosis of patients with CHD and found, in general, a poorer outcome in blacks.[15] Unfortunately, the pathways through which such social and cultural factors are operative are not fully understood.[17]

Physician factors

The primary caregiver – most often the physician – is felt to be of foremost importance in the successful implementation of preventive services. Barriers at this level are many, as constraints on time and resources are great.

Many practitioners are aware of current recommendations for lipid lowering but do not appreciate the magnitude of the benefits, especially when compared with aggressive interventional management.[18] Physicians may also lack confidence in their own ability to effectively implement a cholesterol-lowering regimen, be it diet or pharmacological therapy.[19,20] One reason for this may be that medical training is focused on treating manifest disease and not preventing disease. Both in medical school and in residency training, learning is hospital-based and geared to acute illness.

Not surprisingly, physicians have not made preventive services a priority. Boekeloo et al. surveyed medical housestaff and attending physicians at Johns Hopkins Hospital with regard to their knowledge, attitudes, and practice patterns of cholesterol management.[21] These medical staff were asked how often a number of barriers kept them from intervening on elevated cholesterol levels. Housestaff cited patient inattentiveness to lifestyle counseling, lack of time to counsel, time demands to focus on the acute illness, and lack of skills in behavior modification as important barriers; attending physicians cited their consulting role without primary care responsibility as a major problem.[21]

Danielsson and Aberg examined physicians' attitudes to and management of hyperlipidemia 18 months after the publication of Swedish national guidelines.[22] They sent a questionnaire to three groups of physicians: primary health practitioners; occupational physicians; and physicians based in internal medicine departments in hospitals. Cholesterol screening was carried out by 15 percent of the primary practitioners, by 65 percent of the occupational physicians, and by 9 percent of the hospital-based physicians. The question 'Is it important to know your blood lipid values?' was answered 'Yes' by 57 percent of the primary practitioners, by 66 percent of occupational, and by 52 percent of hospital-based physicians. The authors comment that agreeing with guidelines does not necessarily bring about change in behavior, and that discussion of physician attitude as well as knowledge is important.[22] A later investigation by McBride et al. reviewed the medical records of 603 patients with CHD who were aged between 27 and 70 years and who were drawn from 45 practices in four states. It was found that 33 percent of patients were not screened with lipid panels, 45 percent did not receive dietary counseling, and 67 percent were not receiving lipid-lowering medication.[23]

Another issue is who should be responsible for risk factor management – the cardiologist, the primary care physician, or the allied health professional? Cardiologists have not, in general, been specifically trained in lipid management.[20] As previously discussed, this results in either no or inadequate lipid treatment; treatment may be taken on by other specialties, such as endocrinologists, and may fragment care. In addition, cardiologists are trained and reimbursed for procedures (both non-invasive and interventional), and have not been trained in billing for preventive services. When hospitalized for treatment of acute myocardial infarction (MI), patients may not receive risk factor management by the cardiologist. When they are subsequently seen by their primary care physician, this in turn may suggest to the generalist that interventions to treat lipid abnormalities are not important.[24]

Organizational barriers: healthcare settings

The hospital poses particular barriers to the provision of preventive services. Yet in this acute setting, the patient may be more receptive to modifying behavior and beginning therapies. Factors which relate in particular to healthcare settings are listed in Box 10.1, p.160: acute care priority, lack of resources and facilities, lack of systems for preventive services, and time and economic constraints.[7]

Societal and health system factors

A major barrier that currently exists is the requirement by many health maintenance organizations or managed care plans that any preventive intervention demonstrates a short-term payoff. This has persisted despite recent primary and secondary prevention trials that show reduced morbidity and mortality.

STRATEGIES TO IMPROVE IMPLEMENTATION

Interventions by physicians

PHYSICIAN EDUCATION PROGRAMS

Training programs for cardiovascular specialists should include modification of risk factors, both pharmacological and non-pharmacological, and also knowledge of the pathophysiology that supports lipid reduction (i.e. vascular biology). Although continuing medical education (CME) programs in the United States are widespread, their impact on physician performance and patient outcome remains unclear.[25,26] In a report by Browner et al., physician compliance with recommendations of the NCEP was not improved by intensive CME.[27] More interactive interventions, such as reminders to physicians, medical record audits, and individualized feedback, are more likely to be effective.[18]

CONSENSUS STATEMENTS/GUIDELINES

Many sets of guidelines and consensus statements have been issued during the past decade regarding the detection and treatment of hyperlipidemia. The impact of these documents remains uncertain,[29] and often conflicting opinions are put forth. Hill et al. have shown that while awareness of guidelines may be as high as 60 percent within 1 year of release, actual compliance may be quite low.[30] Adherence also depends on the group issuing a set of guidelines and the target audience. For example, in one review, 80 percent of cardiologists were aware of the American College of Cardiology guidelines for exercise testing; this contrasted with 29 percent awareness for those issued by the American College of Physicians.[31] Lomas et al. concluded that without incentives, or removal of disincentives, guidelines were not likely to change actual clinical practice,[29] while Giles et al. conducted telephone interviews of 154 735 adults to assess trends in the percentage of patients treated for high cholesterol by a physician. The percentage increased from 7.6 to 11.7 percent (p < 0.001) over 2 years, though the authors believe that some of this increase may be due to dissemination of NCEP-ATP guidelines that were mailed to primary care physicians.[3]

Schucker et al. reported on National Heart, Lung, and Blood Institute-sponsored national telephone surveys of practicing physicians and the adult public in 1983, 1986, and 1990 to assess attitudes and practices regarding high serum cholesterol.[32] Over this time period there were several educational efforts proposed, such as the NCEP guidelines, as well as public campaigns. In 1990, physicians reported treating cholesterol at considerably lower blood levels than in 1983 or 1986. The number of adults who reported having had their cholesterol checked rose from 35 to 65 percent between 1983 and 1990, and medication use increased from 3 percent to 9 percent during the same period. These changes suggest educational gains; the data also suggest areas for continued cholesterol educational initiatives.[32]

Headrick et al. compared three approaches for improving compliance with the practice guidelines of the NCEP.[33] A control group of physicians received only the standard lecture, a second group had lecture and generic chart reminders, while a third group had lecture plus patient-specific feedback and explicit recommendations. Knowledge of lipid disorders was tested before and after, and attitudes were surveyed following intervention. Despite the labor-intensive efforts in the third group, improvements were modest and they were not significantly related to the lecture attendance or physician knowledge.

Unfortunately, different professional groups have issued guidelines with conflicting recommendations. One example is the guidelines for detection of hyperlipidemia issued by the American College of Physicians (ACP)[34] and the NCEP ATP II.[35] The ACP guidelines are markedly more conservative; for example, they recommend screening for lipid abnormalities only in men aged between 35 and 65 years, and in women aged between 45 and 65, using only total cholesterol. The ATP II states that everyone aged 20 years and older should have their total cholesterol, as well as high-density lipoprotein-cholesterol (HDL-C) measured in the initial screening. Significant numbers of patients at risk would be missed using ACP guidelines. This may not necessarily be patients who require drug therapy, but those who deserve identification of elevated lipids for diet therapy and more frequent monitoring.[36]

PERFORMANCE FEEDBACK

Feedback can have an impact on physician performance. Most feedback has been based on medical record audits, personalized written communication, computer-generated feedback and one-on-one discussion. In general, the more personalized the feedback, the greater impact on physician performance.[28]

Interventions by allied health professionals

A multidisciplinary approach to preventive care in general – and treatment of hyperlipidemia in particular – is ideal for successful implementation. As discussed earlier, physicians are not trained in many aspects of preventive care, and time restraints limit discussion with patient as well as careful follow-up.

NURSE CASE-MANAGEMENT PROGRAMS

The organizational and staffing barriers to implementation of preventive services can, in part, be overcome using nurse case-managers. They have been shown to be cost-effective and to provide excellent continuity between inpatient and ambulatory care settings for management of many risk factors, including lipid lowering.[37] In a randomized trial of nurse case-manager program versus usual care, DeBusk et al. demonstrated a significantly higher rate of smoking cessation and a tripling of the proportion of patients reaching the LDL-C goal of 100 mg/dL or less among those patients managed by specially trained nurses.[38] Nurse case-managers seem to be especially effective in increasing adherence to diet and drugs.[7] Case-manager telephone contacts with patients provide an important measure of surveillance, instruction, and support.

NURSING EDUCATION PROGRAMS

Programs exist to train nurses in the management of hyperlipidemia (NCEP for Nurses), though many who undergo this training do not have the opportunity to utilize their skills in the current hospital or ambulatory care setting.

NURSING STANDARDS/CLINICAL GUIDELINES

Nursing standards and guidelines for risk factor modification have not yet been adequately developed. This may be in part due to lack of a defined role and reimbursement for nurses to perform these services. Problems in implementing guidelines appear to be similar to those for physicians.

Interventions in healthcare institutions (hospitals, clinics, practices)

Initiation of preventive care can ideally be undertaken in the hospital setting. A study examining cholesterol management in patients undergoing coronary bypass surgery found that nearly half of the patients admitted for surgery had elevated cholesterol levels and of these, half were unaware of this.[39] The authors propose that rehabilitation programs that are begun during hospitalization are ideal for management of hypercholesterolemia because many patients may make initial changes but fail to sustain them when they are not acutely sick or when they are feeling better. This also gives nurses an opportunity to work with patients for education and feedback.

IDENTIFICATION OF PATIENTS

This can be undertaken by laboratories, clinical units, or nurse-generated forms. Cholesterol values identified as abnormal by laboratory computers are more likely to lead to follow-up treatment than those that are not so labeled.[40]

REFERRAL CLINICS WITH SUBSPECIALTY SERVICES

There is ongoing controversy – both in the medical literature and by healthcare reformers – about who is best able to treat a variety of medical problems. Some studies have shown that cardiovascular specialists are uniquely suited to treat cardiovascular problems, provide better treatment, and reduce overall costs.[41]

Specialized laboratories are often required in the work-up of a patient with lipid abnormalities. Blood tests that are carried out in conjunction with detection and treatment of hyperlipidemia often require specialized testing that must be undertaken in a standardized laboratory. If such a facility is not available at a particular site, then samples should be sent to such a laboratory.

Interventions in healthcare systems and third-party payors

HEALTHCARE SYSTEMS

Hospitals must facilitate provision of preventive services. As discussed earlier, this includes staff and system organization that is given time and training to provided these patient services. This can take the form of physicians and trainees or nurse practitioners. In addition, specialty clinics can be set up for patient referral.

As an increasing amount of patient care is determined by managed care, it is imperative that primary and secondary prevention be recognized. In the Health Plan Employer Data Information Set it states that managed care will get behind the effort to control cholesterol in patients with known coronary artery disease.[42]

REIMBURSEMENT POLICIES

This is perhaps one of the greatest deterrents to implementation of preventive care. The lack of reimbursement can serve as a powerful disincentive to risk factor management by the practicing physician.[43,44] This absence of reimbursement reinforces efforts toward acute care services and intervention.

The cost-effectiveness of cholesterol-lowering drugs has been demonstrated. In general, it appears that these medicines may be relatively cost-effective depending on the specific group of patients, the drug used, patient age and sex, the presence of vascular disease, and the risk factor profile.[45]

A cost-effectiveness analysis by Prosser et al. showed that secondary prevention with a statin was cost-effective for all sub-groups, and was even cost-saving in some high-risk sub-groups.[46] Statin drugs for primary prevention may not be cost-effective for those at low risk, however.

The cost-effectiveness in older patients (age >75 years) with previous MI has been demonstrated, although there is not agreement in this area. An analysis of published data by Glanz et al. found that statin therapy appeared as cost-effective as many other routinely accepted medical interventions in these patients.[47]

Johannesson et al. analyzed the cost-effectiveness of simvastatin to lower blood cholesterol levels using data from the Scandinavian Simvastatin Survival Study (4S).[48] In this study, simvastatin was shown to reduce overall mortality in patients with pre-existing CHD. Excluding indirect costs (i.e. for lost production), the direct costs for each year of life gained ranged from $3800 for a 70-year-old man with total cholesterol of 309 mg/dL to $27 400 for a 35-year-old woman with total cholesterol of 213 mg/dL. The cost-effectiveness of population-wide approaches to treating hyperlipidemia was estimated using the Coronary Heart Disease Policy Model; this is a computer-based model with projections based on the assumption that data from clinical trials can be applied broadly. The authors found that a cost of $4.95 per person per year would lower cholesterol by 2 percent, and would prolong life at an estimated cost of $320 per year of life saved. This compares favorably with many other accepted medical interventions.

In a discussion of provision of preventive services in the changing healthcare system, Pearson et al. concluded that a system in which each person has access to a primary care provider should have striking effects on the provision of preventive services.[49] These authors also cite data suggesting that preventive care behavior of lower socioeconomic groups may not change without considerable additional outreach and educational efforts despite changes in access to primary care.[10]

LEGISLATION AND REGULATION

Preventive care is increasingly becoming part of national agendas, though how this will translate into practice has yet to be determined. One example is the New York State Hospital-Based Coronary Prevention Program, where as part of a Certificate of Need application for initiation or expansion of cardiac surgical or invasive cardiologic services, hospitals in New York State are required to submit a preventive cardiology plan for risk factor identification and management in patients with coronary disease.

MEDICAL–LEGAL ACTIONS

Recent medical-legal actions may be another example of use of quality assurance standards. A recently settled suit, successfully charging a wrongful death due in part to the lack of treatment of hyperlipidemia, illustrates the use of guidelines in medical malpractice claims.[50]

Pharmacological issues

The development of new lipid-lowering agents and new formulations of existing drugs continues. These drugs are generally taken for a lifetime and therefore represent a very good investment for pharmaceutical companies. The development of once-daily medications with few side effects is reflected in lower discontinuation rates and greater patient compliance.[9]

Recommendations

Risk factor management in general – and treatment of dyslipidemias in particular – has now been demonstrated in both primary and secondary prevention of CHD. Unfortunately, for all of our technical advances in diagnosis and treatment of CHD, we have not made equal progress in prevention. This chapter has outlined the extent of the problem and proposed several strategies that will enable us to better serve our patients. An editorial by Brown and Goldstein in *Science*, 'Heart Attacks: Gone with the Century' states that better understanding and treatment of cholesterol may well end coronary disease as a major public health problem early in the next century.[51] However, a great many studies need to be carried out in order to fulfil this promise.

REFERENCES

1. National Health and Nutrition Examination Survey III (NHANES III). National Center for Health Statistics, Centers for Disease Control and Prevention, 1994. Unpublished data.
2. Sempos C, Fulwood R, Haines C, *et al*. The prevalence of high blood cholesterol levels among adults in the United States. *JAMA* 1989; **262**: 45–52.
3. Giles WH, Anda RF, Jones DH, Serdula MK, Merritt RK, DeStefano F. Recent trends in the identification and treatment of high blood cholesterol by physicians. *JAMA* 1993; **269**: 1133–8.
4. Marcelino JJ, Feingold KR. Inadequate treatment with HMG-CoA reductase inhibitors by health care providers. *Am J Med* 1996; **100**: 605–10.
5. Pearson TA, Kris-Etherton PM, Shannon BM, Lewis C, Jenkins LK. Attainment of low density lipoprotein (LDL) cholesterol goals in primary care practice: success depends on baseline level of risk. *Circulation* 1996; **94**: 702–13.
6. ASPIRE Steering Group. A British Cardiac Society survey of the potential for the secondary prevention of coronary disease: ASPIRE (Action in Second Prevention through Intervention to Reduce Events). Principal Results. *Heart* 1996; **75**: 334–42.
7. Pearson TA, McBride PE, Miller NH, Smith SC. Task Force 8: Organization of Preventive Cardiology Service. *J Am Coll Cardiol* 1996; **27**: 964–1047.

8. Kottke TE, Brekke ML, Solbert LI. Making time for preventive services. *Mayo Clin Proc* 1993; **68**: 785–91.

9. Simons LA, Levis G, Simons J. Apparent discontinuation rates in patients prescribed lipid-lowering drugs. *Med J Aust* 1996; **164**: 208–11.

10. Andrade SE, Walker AM, Gottlieb LK, Hollenberg NK, Testa MA, Soperia GM, Platt R. Discontinuation of antihyperlipidemic drugs – do rates reported in clinical trials reflect rates in primary care settings? *N Engl J Med* 1995; **332**: 1125–31.

11. Avorn J, Monette J, Lacour A, Bohn RL, Monane M, Mogun H, Lelorier J. Persistence of use of lipid-lowering medications. *JAMA* 1998; **279**: 1458–62.

12. Schectman G, Hiatt J. Drug therapy for hypercholesterolemia in patients with cardiovascular disease: factors limiting achievement of lipid goals. *Am J Med* 1996; **100**: 197–204.

13. Kaplan GA, Keil JE. Socioeconomic factors and cardiovascular disease: a review of the literature. *Circulation* 1995; **88**: 1973–98.

14. Williams RE, Barefoot JC, Califf RM, *et al*. Prognostic importance of social and economic resources among medically treated patients with angiographically defined coronary heart disease. *JAMA* 1992; **267**: 520–4.

15. Castaner A, Simmons BE, Mar M, Cooper R. Myocardial infarction in black patients: poor prognosis after hospital discharge. *Ann Intern Med* 1988; **109**: 33–5.

16. Tofler GH, Stone PH, Muller JE, *et al*. Effects of gender and race on prognosis after myocardial infarction: adverse prognosis in women, particularly black women. *J Am Coll Cardiol* 1987; **9**: 473–82.

17. Lenfant C. Conference on socioeconomic status and cardiovascular health and disease. *Circulation* 1996; **94**: 2041–4.

18. Yogel RA. Comparative clinical consequences of aggressive lipid management, coronary angioplasty, and bypass surgery in coronary artery disease. *Am J Cardiol* 1992; **69**: 1229–33.

19. Shea S, Gemson DH, Mossel P. Management of high blood cholesterol by primary care physicians: diffusion of the National Cholesterol Education Program Adult Treatment Panel guidelines. *J Gen Intern Med* 1990; **5**: 327–34.

20. Roberts WC. Getting cardiologists interested in lipids. *Am J Cardiol* 1993; **72**: 744–5.

21. Boekeloo, B, Becker DM, LeBailly A, Pearson TA. Cholesterol management in patients hospitalized for coronary heart disease. *Am J Prev Med* 1988; **4**: 128–32.

22. Danielsson B, Aberg H. Hyperlipidemia – management and views amongst physicians in general practice, in occupational health care, and in internal medicine. *J Intern Med* 1993; **234**: 411–16.

23. McBride P, Schrott HG, Plane MB, Underbakke G, Brown RL. Primary care practice adherence to national cholesterol education program guidelines for patients with coronary heart disease. *Arch Intern Med* 1998; **158**: 1238–44.

24. Boekeloo B, Becker D, Yeo E, Pearson T A, Gillian R. Post-myocardial infarction cholesterol management by primary physicians (abstract). *J Am Coll Cardiol* 1995; **25**: 77A.

25. Haynes RB, Davis DA, McKibbon A, Tugwell P. A critical appraisal of the efficacy of continuing medical education. *JAMA* 1984; **251**: 61–4.

26. Stein LS. The effectiveness of continuing medical education: eight research reports. *J Med Educ* 1981; **65**: 103–10.

27. Browner WS, Baron RB, Solkowitz S, Adler LJ, Gullion DS. Physician management of hypercholesterolemia. A randomized trail of continuing medical education. *West J Med* 1994; **161**: 572–8.

28. Davis AA, Thompson MA, Oxman AA, Haynes RB. Changing physician performance. A systematic review of the effect of continuing medical education strategies. *JAMA* 1995; **274**: 700–5.

29. Lomas J, Anderson GM, Domnick-Pierre K, Vayda E, Enkin MW, Hannah WI. Do practice guidelines guide practice? The effect of a consensus statement on the practice of physicians. *N Engl J Med* 1989; **321**: 1306–11.

30. Hill MN, Levine DM, Whelton PK. Awareness, use, and impact of the 1984 Joint National Committee consensus report on high blood pressure. *Am J Public Health* 1988; **78**: 1190–4.

31. Tunis SR, Hayward RS, Wilson MC, *et al.* Internists' attitudes about clinical practice guidelines. *Ann Intern Med* 1994; **120**: 956–63.

32. Schucker B, Wittes JT, Santanello NC, Weber SJ, McGoldrick D, Donato K, Levy A, Rifkin BM. Change in cholesterol awareness and action. *Arch Intern Med* 1991; **151**: 666–73.

33. Headrick LA, Speroff T, Pelecanos HI, Cebul RD. Efforts to improve compliance with the national cholesterol educational program guidelines. *Arch Intern Med* 1992; **152**: 2490–6.

34. Garber AM, Browner WS. American College of Physicians guidelines for using serum cholesterol, high-density lipoprotein cholesterol, and triglycerides as screening tests for the prevention of coronary heart disease in adults. *Ann Intern Med* 1996; **124**: 515–17.

35. National Cholesterol Education Program. Second Report of the Expert Panel on detection, evaluation, and treatment of high cholesterol in adults (Adult Treatment Panel II). *Circulation* 1994; **89**: 1329–445.

36. Myerson M, Lewis C, Jenkins PL, Nichols M, Pearson TA. Cholesterol screening according to the American College of Physicians (ACP) guidelines: who is missed? (Abstract). *J Am Coll Cardiol* 1997; **29** (Suppl. A): 226A.

37. Blair TP, Bryant FJ, Bocuzzi S. Treatment of hypercholesterolemia by a clinical nurse using a stepped-care protocol in a non-volunteer population. *Arch Intern Med* 1988; **148**: 1046–8.

38. DeBusk RF, Houston-Miller N, Superko HR, *et al.* A case-management system for coronary risk factor modification after acute myocardial infarction. *Ann Intern Med* 1994; **120**: 721–9.

39. Watt P, Becker DM, Salaita, Pearson TA. Hypercholesterolemia in patients undergoing coronary bypass surgery: Are they aware, under treatment, and under control? *Heart Lung* 1988; **17**: 205–8.

40. Reed RG, Jenkins PL, Pearson TA. Laboratory's manner of reporting serum cholesterol affects clinical care. *Clin Chem* 1994; **40**: 847–8.

41. Jollis JG, DeLong ER, Peterson ED, Muhlbaier LB, Fortin DF, Califf RM, Mark DB. Outcome of acute myocardial infarction according to the specialty of the admitting physician. *N Engl J Med* 1996; **335**: 1880–7.

42. National Committee for Quality Assurance 1999. HEDIS 1999 update to Volume I: Narrative March 1999, Annapolis MD.

43. Eisenberg JM. Physician utilization. The state of research about physicians' practice patterns. *Med Care* 1985; **23**: 461–83.

44. Taylor RB. Health promotion: Can it succeed in the office? *Prev Med* 1981; **10**: 258–62.

45. Hamilton VH, Raccicot F-E, Zowall H, Coupal L, Grover SA. The cost-effectiveness of HMG-CoA reductase inhibitors to prevent coronary heart disease. *JAMA* 1995; **273**: 1032–8.

46. Prosser LA, Stinnett AA, Goldman P A, Williams L W, Hunink MGM, Goldman L, Weinstein MC. Cost-effectiveness of cholesterol-lowering therapies according to selected patient characteristics. *Ann Intern Med* 2000; **132**: 769–79.

47. Glanz DA, Kuntz KM, Jacobson G, Avorn J. Cost-effectiveness of 3-hydroxy-3-methylglutaryl coenzyme A reductase inhibitor therapy in older patients with myocardial infarction. *Ann Intern Med* 2000; **132**: 780–7.

48. Johannesson M, Jonsson B, Kjekshus J, Olsson AG, Pederson TR, Wedel H. Cost-effectiveness of simvastatin treatment to lower cholesterol levels in patients with coronary heart disease. *N Engl J Med* 1997; **336**: 332–6.

49. Pearson TA, Spencer M, Jenkins P. Who will provide preventive services? *J Public Health Management Practice* 1995; **1**: 16–27.

50. Woman's death leads to award by jurors. *The Oregonian*, May 1, 1996.

51. Brown MS, Goldstein JL. 'Heart Attacks: gone with the Century?' Editorial. *Science* 1996; **72**: 629.

11

Report of the Adult Treatment Panel III (ATP III): The 2001 National Cholesterol Education Program (NCEP) guidelines on the detection evaluation and treatment of elevated cholesterol in adults

RICHARD C PASTERNAK

INTRODUCTION

Cholesterol guidelines for the adult United States population have been updated and released by the National Heart Lung and Blood Institute.[1,2] The report of the Adult Treatment Panel III (ATP III) contains updated clinical guidelines for lipid testing and management in adults; as such, it is the most recent component of the National Cholesterol Education Program (NCEP) which itself began during the late 1980s. There have been two previous panel guideline reports for adult treatment, and others that have addressed aspects of cholesterol measurement and management (including population recommendations, laboratory guidelines, and standards for the treatment of children and adolescents).

As busy clinicians know, the past one to two decades have seen clinical guidelines increasingly become part of the daily life of practicing medicine. The importance of such guidelines can be tracked to at least two developments that are likely responsible for the emergence of guidelines: first, practice is now increasingly 'evidence-based' medicine; and second, contemporary medical management has become even more complex. As our understanding of the complexity of lipid metabolism has increased, we have been presented with a wider array of laboratory tests and pharmacological interventions. There have now been tens of thousands of patients enrolled in primary and secondary prevention trials of lipid active drugs (largely statins) demonstrating the benefit of medical intervention.[3] Numerous smaller supplementary studies have focused on specific sub-groups and on atherosclerosis progression. Together, this work documents clear effectiveness of lipid active therapies.

Guidelines, for cholesterol and other issues, are often simultaneously criticized both for their complexity *and* their oversimplification of management. Clinically simple problems do not need guidelines. Ideally, guidelines interpret and compile complex information to present the information in a simplified format. The challenge is to present inherently complex issues in a clinically useful format. Guidelines have come to have a greater role in daily practice in large part because of the increasing complexity of medical management, and the greater time pressures in the era of managed care. Despite medical advances, these complexities and time pressures are largely responsible for a widely documented gap between the recommendations contained in clinical guidelines and the application and implementation of these guidelines.[4] In fact, largely because of this treatment gap, the NCEP held off delivering new cholesterol guidelines while working hard to improve the gap. By the late 1990s, however, it had become clear that the importance of new information available from recent trials made it imperative that new guidelines be developed and released. It was also recognized that new insights regarding implementation – particularly for lifestyle changes – made it important to include that information in a new report.

ATP III was chaired by Scott M. Grundy, MD PhD, assisted by ex-official members from the NHLBI staff, and by several consultants. Drafts underwent sequential reviews by more than 20 outside senior expert reviewers, and by the full Coordinating Committee of NCEP. An executive summary of the final report, released on May 15, 2001, and the full report, are available on the NHLBI/NCEP website. (www.nhlbi.nih.gov/guidelines/cholesterol).

NEW FEATURES OF ATP III

When the full ATPIII report is compared with the previous reports issued in 1993 and 1988, a new approach is immediately evident. The full report includes a series of 'evidence statements,' aligned to specific evidence-based 'recommendations.' The evidence is classified by *type*, and includes four categories: (A) Major randomized controlled clinical trials; (B) smaller controlled trials and meta-analyses; (C) observational and metabolic studies; and (D) clinical experience. The evidence is then rated by strength: '1' if it was felt by the panel to be 'very strong'; '2' if it was felt to be 'moderately strong'; and '3' if it was felt to show a 'strong trend.'

Numerous references (over 1200 in total) support the evidence and evidence statements.

Recommendations from ATP III begin with the requirement of a complete lipid profile for all patients aged 20 years or older. Lipid and lipoprotein classifications have also been modified:

- LDL of <100 mg/dL is defined as 'optimal' for the entire population.
- Low HDL as a categorical risk factor has been raised from <35 mg/dL to <40 mg/dL, and there are lower triglyceride classification cutpoints (normal <150 mg/dL), with more attention to moderate elevations.

While LDL-cholesterol (LDL-C) remains the primary target for these patients, once the LDL target has been achieved, then a 'non-HDL-cholesterol (HDL-C)' target is also specified for individuals with triglycerides between 200 and 499 mg/dL. Non-HDL-C is calculated as follows:

$$\text{Non-HDL-C} = \text{total cholesterol} - \text{HDL-C}.$$

Interventions termed 'therapeutic lifestyle changes' (TLC) receive considerable attention in ATP III, shifting the focus from dietary 'steps' and general advice on physical activity to a much more comprehensive review of effective lifestyle interventions for a full range of patient types. The use of plant stanols/sterols (2 g per day) and soluble fiber (10–25 g per day) has been added to the dietary recommendations, and there is particular emphasis on weight management as well as physical activity (Table 11.1).

Table 11.1 *NCEP-ATP III lifestyle diet. Nutrient composition of the Therapeutic Lifestyle Changes (TLC) diet*

Nutrient	Recommended intake
Saturated fat[a]	<7% of total calories
Polyunsaturated fat	Up to 10% of total calories
Monounsaturated fat	Up to 20% of total calories
Total fat	25–35% of total calories
Carbohydrate[b]	50–60% of total calories
Fiber	20–30 g per day
Protein	Approximately 15% of total calories
Cholesterol	<200 mg per day
Total calories[c]	Balanced energy intake and expenditure to maintain desirable body weight/prevent weight gain

[a] *Trans* fatty acids are another LDL – raising fat that should be kept at a low intake.
[b] Carbohydrates should be derived predominantly from foods rich in complex carbohydrates including grains, especially whole grains, fruits, and vegetables.
[c] Daily energy expenditure should include at least moderate physical activity (contributing approximately 200 kcal per day).

The ATP III report focuses attention on the concept of risk and risk assessment, considering 'long-term' or lifetime risk, as well as 'short-term' or 10-year risk. Lifetime or long-term risk is important in people at relatively low shorter-term risk, but who have a single dominant risk factor. This report indicates the importance of recognizing healthy individuals with abnormalities of even one risk factor. While recognizing that it is clearly appropriate to focus more intensive risk lowering strategies (especially drug therapies) on individuals at higher short-term (10-year) levels of risk, individuals with higher lifetime risk are candidates for more intensive therapeutic lifestyle interventions.

The 1996 American College of Cardiology 27th Bethesda Conference[5] began to popularize the importance concept, embedded in previous NCEP reports, that a basic principle of prevention recognizes the need to match the intensity of risk-reducing interventions to the level of risk. In particular, ATP III provides for the identification and management of persons at high absolute risk without clinically evident atherosclerotic disease. A key high-risk group without evident vascular disease includes patients with diabetes. The multiple risk factor abnormalities present in diabetics places them at very high risk for future coronary heart disease (CHD) events. Also, diabetics who develop CHD have higher mortality and morbidity than age-matched non-diabetic patients.[6]

A second new high-risk group in ATP III includes patients whose 10-year CHD risk is ≥20 percent by using Framingham global risk scoring. These two groups (diabetics and patients with a ≥20% CHD 10-year risk) are considered to be 'CHD risk equivalents,' as their 10-year-risk is 'equivalent' to the 10-year-risk of an individual with stable CHD.

The final high-risk group receiving special attention in ATP III are patients with the 'metabolic syndrome' (Table 11.2). Patients with multiple metabolic abnormalities may have varying absolute 10-year CHD risk; nevertheless, such patients are at clearly increased risk. Furthermore, their risk can be markedly attenuated by intensified therapeutic lifestyle changes, particularly weight reduction and increased physical activity.

To estimate the 10-year risk, the Framingham investigators have developed a sophisticated mathematical model[7,8] that integrates age, gender, total cholesterol, systolic blood pressure, HDL-cholesterol, smoking status, and the presence and levels of multiple clinical risk factors into a prediction model. From this model, one estimates the absolute risk (as a percentage) that any given individual will develop a 'hard' CHD event (myocardial infarction or cardiac death). This risk estimation model allows both professionals and the public rapidly to calculate an individual's 10-year risk. This 10-year risk score can also serve as a motivational tool for both providers and patients, in order to help individuals to focus on lowering of risk factors so that overall risk will be lowered. One calculates risk through the use of a variety of NCEP-produced documents, a paper version, a web-based version of the scoring system, a spreadsheet downloaded onto a personal computer from the NCEP website, a similar program downloaded to a palm-held device, or a paper version of the scoring system.

Finally, the ATP III report also devotes considerable attention to the importance of adherence to the recommendations contained in these prevention guidelines. As already noted, there is considerable evidence of poor adherence to guidelines by both individuals and providers. The large benefits seen in clinical trials can only be

Table 11.2 *Clinical identification of the metabolic syndrome*

Risk factor	Defining level[a]
Abdominal obesity[b] (waist circumference)[c]	
Men	>102 cm (>40 in)
Women	>88 cm (>35 in)
Triglycerides	≥150 mg/dL
HDL-cholesterol	
Men	<40 mg/dL
Women	<50 mg/dL
Blood pressure	≥130/≥85 mmHg
Fasting glucose	≥110 mg/dL

[a]An individual needs to have three or more of the five features listed to have the diagnosis of metabolic syndrome.
[b]Overweight and obesity are associated with insulin resistance and the metabolic syndrome. However, the presence of abdominal obesity is more highly correlated with the metabolic risk factors than is an elevated body mass index (BMI). Therefore, the simple measure of waist circumference is recommended to identify the body weight component of the metabolic syndrome.
[c]Some male patients can develop multiple metabolic risk factors when the waist circumference is only marginally increased, e.g. 94–102 cm (37–40 in). Such patients may have strong genetic contribution to insulin resistance and they should benefit from changes in life habits, similarly to men with categorical increases in waist circumference.

achieved in practice if adherence to interventions used in these trials occurs at a rate similar to that achieved in the clinical trials. By detailing solutions to the 'treatment gap,' ATP III hopes to improve this problem. The report includes a comprehensive review of behavioral medicine, practice pattern, and public health literature. It also suggests state-of-the-art multidisciplinary strategies for targeting the patient, clinicians, and health delivery systems, in order to achieve more effective implementation of these new guidelines.

CONCLUSIONS

The ATP III report represents an important advance from previous ATP reports dating back to the late 1980s. The guidelines are more tightly evidence-based than previous reports, partly due to the evolution of the guideline process, requiring clearly delineated links between evidence and recommendations, and also because of the robust evidence base published over the past decade. An important change in ATP III is the expansion of the high-risk category to include patients without evident vascular disease, but with a level of risk equivalent to those patients with established CHD. This group, termed 'coronary heart disease equivalents,' now includes patients with diabetes, and those with a 10-year absolute risk of over 20 percent for CHD events. With the ATP III report, the Framingham risk score is formally introduced into the guideline process. The scoring system allows for easy calculation of the absolute risk for an individual of having a 'hard' CHD event (myocardial infarction, or CHD death). The report also discusses in detail concepts of lifetime or long-term risk. ATP III has broadened recommendations for lifestyle change termed 'therapeutic lifestyle change' (TLC), and eliminated the step 1 and step 2 diet approach. Finally, the report details established approaches to improve adherence and provides patients and clinicians with a set of implementation tools to enhance use of the guidelines and compliance with the guidelines' recommendations. It is hoped that by improved understanding, recognition of a firm evidence base, and education through multiple channels, that adherence with the new ATP III guidelines will improve the care of our population by more effectively targeting lipid factors which lead to the development and progression of atherosclerotic cardiovascular disease.

ATP III at-a-glance: the report in nine steps

The NCEP has provided a nine-step version of ATP III termed 'ATP III at-a-glance: quick desk reference.' This document is available in print, as well as web-based, or palm OS interactive versions. These straightforward steps attempt to simplify the complex issues addressed in ATP III and provide a useful guide for the busy clinician.

REFERENCES

1. Expert Panel on Detection, Evaluation, and Treatment of High Blood Cholesterol in Adults. Executive Summary of the third report of the National Cholesterol Education Program (NCEP) expert panel on detection, evaluation, and treatment of high blood cholesterol in adults (Adult Treatment Panel III). *JAMA* 2001; **285**: 2486–97.
2. Third report of the National Cholesterol Education Program (NCEP) expert panel on detection, evaluation, and treatment of high blood cholesterol in adults (Adult Treatment Panel III). Final Report. *Circulation* 2002; **106**: 3145–3421.
3. Larosa JC, He J, Vupputuri S. Effects of statins on risk of coronary disease. A meta-analysis of randomized controlled trials. 1999; **282**: 2340–6.
4. Pearson TA, Laurora I, Chu H, Kafonek S. The lipid treatment assessment project (L-TAP): a multicenter survey to evaluate the percentages of dyslipidemic patients receiving lipid-lowering therapy and achieving low-density lipoprotein cholesterol goals. *Arch Intern Med* 2000; **160**: 459–67.
5. Pearson TA, Fuster V. Matching the intensity of risk factor management with the hazard for coronary disease events. 27th Bethesda Conference. Executive Summary. *J Am Coll Cardiol* 1996; **27**: 961–3.
6. Haffner SM, Lehto S, Ronnemaa T, Pyorala K, Laakso M. Mortality from coronary heart disease in subjects with type 2 diabetes and in nondiabetic subjects with and without prior myocardial infarction. *N Engl J Med* 1998; **339**: 229–34.
7. Wilson PW, D'Agostino RB, Levy D, *et al*. Prediction of coronary heart disease using risk factor categories. *Circulation* 1998; **97**: 1837–47.
8. Grundy SM, Pasternak R, Greenland P, *et al*. AHA/ACC scientific statement: assessment of cardiovascular risk by use of multiple-risk factor assessment equations: a statement for healthcare professionals from the American Heart Association and the American College of Cardiology. *J Am Coll Cardiol* 1999; **34**: 1348–59.

Index